WHEN FAMILY CALLS

Finding Hope in the Chaos of Long-Distance Caregiving

Caroline H. Sheppard, MSW

BANYAN TREE PRESS

When Family Calls: Finding Hope in the Chaos of Long-Distance Caregiving

ISBN: 978-1-936449-76-7

Cover Design and Interior Layout: Ronda Taylor

Banyan Tree Press

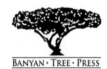
BANYAN · TREE · PRESS

Denver, Colorado
Austin, Texas
www. BanyanTreePress.com

DEDICATION

In loving memory of my father, mother, brother, aunt, and uncle.

CONTENTS

FOREWORD

It is human nature to wonder "what if" this or that would have happened or not have happened at all, to ask why, to want to know what happened to others who experienced what we are about to experience and to discover how they did so well. We seek inspiration and constantly search for new ideas and actions we can take, the "how to" that can make the task in front of us easier. The author's story of her caregiving experiences accomplishes this and more.

Pat Speight, a longtime Irish storyteller was once quoted as saying, "A story is the shortest distance between two people." There is a great deal of truth to this. In this case the author writes in a way that leaves us feeling as if we are physically and emotionally by her side every step of the way as she tries to navigate through a maze of caregiving challenges that, even as a seasoned social worker, were difficult for her. In her introduction she writes, "In my role as caregiver, I found that I used many of the skills I had developed (as a social worker), however many things were completely new to me. Providing care to my own family members tossed me into unknown territory. It was different and not easy."

Her first story is about caring for her father. He suffered from a stroke, numerous medical conditions and eventually dementia. Living at home was not an option. The number of challenges this created was overwhelming at times. After reading about her experiences with her father, I remember thinking to myself what more could I possibly learn by reading about her other experiences with her mother, aunt, uncle and finally her brother. The fact was there was so much more to learn.

Over the past forty years I have spent time with and assisted hundreds of survivors of traumatic incidents including the 1995 bombing of the Federal Building in Oklahoma where 168 people were killed, The Gulf War, the 9/11 Attack On America, Hurricanes Katrina and Rita, the unbelievable killing of young children at Sandy Hook Elementary. I've met with far too many parents of murdered children and friends of those who took their own lives. In my efforts to teach other professionals what matters most in their efforts to help trauma survivors, I found that best lessons came from listening to the stories of these courageous and resilient survivors. In this regard the author does not disappoint us.

There is no better place to discover what others have discovered than in the stories they share with us about their experiences. Each of her stories presents us with new crises, problems and situations we would never imagine could happen. And yes, she walks us through the many ways she dealt with these situations. The journey she takes us on, the stories she tells us compels us to listen. We learn so much from her and need to thank her for bringing us into the world of caregiving with such detail and personal honesty. Her story will help us avoid the missteps, lessen the physical and emotional stress of caregiving and provide us with the support and resources that comes from her sharing the lessons she had to learn firsthand.

Dr. William Steele

Founder, The National Institute for Trauma and Loss in Children (TLC)

INTRODUCTION

From 1999-2014, I cared for five different family members. The need for my help arose quickly, due to aging, critical and chronic illnesses and the surrounding issue of dementia. Like so many others, with one phone call, I became a long distance caregiver, without any preparation or specific training for the "job." I did not live near any of the family members in need, which is not unusual in today's society. This created numerous challenges and complications. I present my caregiving stories chronologically beginning with my father, who suffered a serious stroke that changed his and my mother's life forever. Next I share my mother's individual story after my father died. After his death, my mother lived eight more years with multiple health issues and needs.

While caring for my mother, I kept in close contact with my favorite elderly aunt and uncle, who the year following my mother's passing, faced a sudden crisis due to my uncle breaking his back. They had no children and needed someone to step in quickly to help manage a very complicated life challenge. Until I had to jump on a plane and fly to their home in Michigan, I had no idea how each of their lives were at risk while living alone in their condominium.

Next, while overseeing my aunt and uncle's care, my only brother was diagnosed with colorectal cancer. He had no wife, no children, and no partner to help him in his time of need, which included a host of issues from medical to financial.

For each family member, the layers of problems were unique. My family's illnesses and issues are not uncommon in today's world, yet as I discovered, they can be staggering if not prepared.

Following is a timeline of family crises that began in 1999 and continued through 2014.

October 1999: Father has a major stroke in Michigan

November-December 1999: I temporarily move in with my mother while my father rehabilitates.

February 2000: Move my parents to assisted living in, Florida, near where I lived.

June 2001: My father dies.

November 2001: Mother has stroke and can no longer express wants and needs or ambulate. Long term rehab and the need for Nurses' Aides to stay with her in her assisted living apartment.

September 2002: Mother fractures her hip...long term rehabilitation again. Continues to live in assisted living with nurses' aide.

September 2007: Mother moves into Nursing Home

June 2008: Mother dies

October 2009: We move from south Florida to northern Florida.

October 2009: Uncle breaks his back/Aunt left alone not eating or drinking.

October 2009: Move Aunt into respite-assisted living while uncle rehabs; neither able to return to their home. They are without children.

June 2010: Brother diagnosed with colorectal cancer

August 2010: Brother suffers subarachnoid brainbleed. No longer can manage own affairs.

January 2011: Brother dies.

September 2012: Aunt Dies. Uncle remains in nursing home alone in Michigan. No family or friends to visit in the area.

October 2013: Moved uncle to assisted living near my home in FL.

Moved after two nights to the Memory Care Unit; extreme confusion and health issues.

November 2014: Uncle has congestive heart failure…
rushed to emergency.

February 2014: Uncle dies the day I was going to a conference hosted by the Institute for the Ages, for this book
project.

WHEN THE CALL COMES

So many of us enter into the role as a caregiver quickly and without warning and with very little preparation for what lies ahead from the first phone call alerting us of a family member or friend in crisis. I understand that in today's world the long distance factor is more prevalent due to our mobile society, and it is one of the main reasons I decided to share my personal stories with others.

Each phone call that kick-started my involvement as a caregiver was sudden and unexpected and created feelings of panic leading to tremendous stress, along with overwhelming feelings. Each caregiving experience brought new challenges that I know others can learn from, as did I.

I share my personal experiences, not simply to tell about what happened to my family and myself, but to examine what it's like to be a long-distance caregiver and to offer hope and help to others as they struggle with all of the details involved with caregiving from afar.

This is not a "how to manual" but instead offers ideas that come from experience, the greatest teacher. I take a very close look at the emotional hurdles and obstacles that come with the multiple layers of caregiving. I address ways to get over or around resistance on the part of those who need our help the most, our own resistance or fear about helping, the systems and their staffs, (a very common obstacle), and the need to arm ourselves with as much knowledge about the condition we are dealing with, in order to ask the right questions to get the right help at the right time.

Baby boomers, like me, are often faced with similar experiences, which come with so many difficult and critical decisions and a sense of upheaval to one's own life. I am certain that in my stories there will be things you can relate to in some way. Within each story, I provide meaningful reflection, helpful knowledge gained, as well as relevant information and lessons learned stemming from the multitude of obstacles and challenges I faced from A to Z the moment I answered each "call" for help. I provide some helpful references that have helped me, such as books and articles, or information as to how to actually get what you need for your particular situation.

Why Me?

Finally, if you are now, or were ever a caregiver to someone there may be times you ask or asked yourself, why me? I know that I did, on those bad days when it felt like nothing was going right for the people I was trying to help or for myself for that matter.

Each person comes into the role with varying experience, willingness and knowledge. Because of this, it is important to have resources for all of us to get through the process of caregiving. Is it always manageable? Absolutely not. Is knowledge helpful to have going into the role? Absolutely. Is having support from others important to have? Most certainly! Is everyone a born caregiver? No!

Because more and more of us are faced with a more complicated world with respect to medical care, financial management, and daily living needs, we need to keep up with what is needed when someone needs our help. My professional experience and background was helpful but it did not eliminate the personal struggles associated with my sudden leap into my new role as a caregiver. Let me briefly explain what I did learn from my professional experiences, followed by what it did not prepare me for when my family needed my help.

Caregiving Is Different

When I was a young child, my paternal grandparents came for dinner almost every Sunday. One vivid memory that I have about my grandmother was that each time I saw her she would quiz me about what I wanted to be when I grew up. Each time she asked, it was the exact same question, "What do you want to be when you grow up?"

My answer was always, "I want to be a nurse!"

Her follow up question, "Why do you want to be a nurse?"

My consistent reason given, "To help people!"

To my grandmother my answer was the wrong answer each time. She would say things like, "You don't want to be a nurse, because it's a dirty job."

"What do you mean?" I would question.

Her response was to scrunch up her nose and look disgusted and say, "Because they have to touch pooh!"

I will never forget the look on her face as she said this to me. She told me that I should instead become a doctor. My grandmother's comments about what a nurse had to do, not only made me laugh, it made me question my answer. I never became a nurse or a doctor but did choose a career path that involved helping people as a social worker.

My first glimpse into helping people was around the fifth grade, when a small group volunteered to go to downtown Detroit to deliver a home-cooked meal to needy families during the holidays, usually Thanksgiving. I have vivid memories of the sights, smells and sounds and the happiness it seemed to bring to the families we met. This was a special event that I did with my mother, a fond memory that stands out in my mind. In addition, in high school I signed up to tutor students in a low-income area. I found this to be very special and gratifying.

While attending undergraduate school, I decided early on that I wanted to become a social worker or psychologist. I found out early, during my internships in undergraduate school, that I loved working with kids. I decided to pursue a degree in social work. During graduate school, my first internship was in the schools, covering preschool to high school for one year. My second internship was in a community mental health clinic for children and families. I found both experiences to be helpful in giving me what I needed to teach me the skills necessary to land my first job. I didn't have to look far for this first job, as I was hired by the community mental health clinic, where I was interning as soon as I graduated. After five rewarding years there, I was offered a school social worker position, covering elementary to high school. My primary clients were children, but my work also involved helping families and consulting with teachers and administrators. Consultation with other professionals such as school personnel, protective service caseworkers, medical personnel, physical, speech, occupational therapists and psychologists, was at the core of my job as "helper" in the school system.

Much of my social work role in both settings, clinical and schools, involved being an advocate, therapist, or consultant. My professional experience taught me how to research and find the optimal resources or programs for my clients and their families. The one part of my job that I liked best was the process of collaboration on behalf of those needing assistance. Such work involved working with or within systems, such as families, schools, hospitals, governmental or departments of social services. My role was challenging, oftentimes stressful, and always very interesting and rewarding. As it turned out, it prepared me well for when I unexpectedly needed to step in to care for my parents and relatives over a fifteen-year period of time.

When my family members needed my "help" I was not a nurse to them. What they needed was someone they could trust, who could take care of their day-to-day lives. My responsibilities were varied and required consultation with professionals, frequent and necessary interfacing with many systems, such as banks, hospitals, nursing homes, funeral homes, hospice and even airlines and airports. In my role as caregiver, I found that I used many of the skills I had developed in my work but some things were completely new to me. Providing care to my own family members tossed me into unknown territory. It was different and not easy.

What I Faced

My caregiving situations involved health problems related to aging, and illness, with the added difficulties associated with dementia. Each type of dementia was manifested differently, and each experience was affected by varying financial levels, personalities and their abilities to manage their day to day living due to the degree of their incapacity. Accessibility to resources was an issue in all five situations. One of my family members was faced with some very different challenges when he was suddenly diagnosed with cancer at age fifty eight. The variables that complicated his situation made a big difference in my experience with helping him in his time of need.

My social work experience was helpful for sure, but the role of caregiver was different and it was oftentimes overwhelmingly lonely even though I had people who supported me. The upside of being able to be a caregiver was that I felt so fortunate that I was available to help my family and be with them in their time of need and at the end of their lives.

As I wrote this, I realized that helping my family in need was what I was preparing for all along; the most important "job" I could ever have had. Interestingly, I never was able to have any children myself, and as I took on the role of caregiver, I realized that because I wasn't raising my own children, or helping them move into adulthood, I had a much more open schedule and opportunity to step in and help when the need arose. I remember thinking, so this is why I wasn't blessed with children. It left the door wide open for me to help my family.

Each story I tell contains new information about the challenges presented in caring for family. They cover issues surrounding:

- Being combative, irrational and resistant to leaving their home when you know it's a danger to themselves for them to stay in their home,

- Not capable or able to pay bills or remember how to write a check,

- Unable to find documents crucial to their getting financial help,

- Dealing with excruciating pain and unmanageable symptoms,

- Unwilling to give up their car keys when you are afraid they'll kill someone else or themselves,

- Unwilling to talk about their final wishes in order to establish a living will and end of life plan,

- Issues with medication and medical care,

- Conflicts with care managers, doctors and nurses,

- Having to learn about a variety of medical, neurological and psychiatric conditions in order to be sure members were getting the best help from me as well as their caregivers,

- Caring for family members while I lived in another state and there was no one else to help them,

- Being exposed to an array of feelings I never expected within myself or from others,

- Expecting that the care I provided for my first family member would be the same for all, only to be confronted by all new situations with each member, and

- Watching close family members die despite all that I did.

Had I been aware of and prepared for all these challenges, it would have made what I had to do easier, less painful and less stressful for everyone. I hope reading about my experiences will help you when you get the call.

My stories offer hope in the face of despair and a sense of empowerment despite the overwhelming amount of obstacles along the way.

CHAPTER ONE

MY FIRST "CALL"

My first long distance caregiving experience began on Sunday, October 31, 1999, with a typical phone call home to check on my aging parents. At the time, I lived in Florida and my parents in Michigan. It was a Sunday, and our friends from Michigan had just left after their visit with us for the weekend. It was about five o'clock on Halloween. Soon the "trick or treat" kids would be arriving at our door, so I thought I better call my parents before it got any later, or before I forgot to call them.

My mother was seventy-five, my father seventy-nine. The moment my mother answered the phone, I knew that something was terribly wrong.

"Happy Halloween, Mom! How are you?" I asked.

She hesitantly answered, "Well, it's not very happy here."

"Why is that?" I asked.

She replied, "Your father is acting weird."

I asked more questions. What is he doing? What do you mean by "weird"?

Alarms went off in my head. Fourteen years before this fateful phone call, my mother had suffered a closed head injury from a bike accident and was left with some limitations. Given this factor, I was especially concerned and felt overwhelmed with a feeling of panic. My heart raced and I found myself trying to find the right questions to ask my mother. I struggled to figure out what she meant by weird and to learn how long my father had been behaving in a "weird" way.

My mother sounded scared and was reticent to answer my questions. She repeated that he was "just acting weird."

After some persistence I was able to get a few more details. She told me that sometime during the night, he had fallen between the bed and the wall and could not get back up off of the floor. I am not sure when, but he did manage to get up, but he was "different" and could not give himself his insulin shot. This was unusual because my father had been giving himself insulin injections since his mid-fifties. Two days had passed with him not being able to hold the syringe and give himself his injection. I wondered why they hadn't called 911 for help, so I asked my mother and she told me that my dad would not let her call anyone for help.

My poor mother was in a very frightening situation. She felt she had very few choices and was paralyzed with the fear of reaching out to the world for help because of my father's irrational denial and anger.

I asked my mother to put my father on the phone, so I could assess his status as best as possible. He answered some basic questions for me with slowed and deliberate speech. He did not sound like himself, and was obviously trying very hard to cover up that there was something wrong. He claimed that he was "fine." I asked him the date and he told me the date from three days prior. He had clearly lost his sense of time.

I told my father that I was very concerned about him and that he needed medical attention. I then spoke to my mother and told her that I was going to call the local police and ask them to send an ambulance. My first thought was for my mother to hang up and dial 911, but knew my mother could not handle this task. It was clear to me that I needed to take control of the situation, so I did. I felt nervous about making the call as I was going against my father's wishes. The rational side of me took over and I did the right thing, yet my stomach was in a knot and my heart was racing as I made the call to the police station near my parents' home. I couldn't call 911 because I was out of state so dialed the station directly and explained the situation.

After speaking to the police in Michigan, I called my mother back and stayed on the line with her until the ambulance arrived. This time, waiting gave me the chance to ask more questions to get a better idea of the timeline of events. On the outside I remained calm and reassuring and told her what to expect and that I would fly up to Michigan as soon as possible to help them. Inside, I was wound so tight I felt as though I would burst. Once the ambulance arrived I hung up the phone and told my husband what had happened. He immediately began looking for flights to Detroit.

My Father Couldn't Tie His Shoes

My source of information as to when and what happened to my father came first from my mother, followed by his tennis partners. She was able to tell me that two of my dad's tennis partners brought him home from his Saturday morning doubles tennis game. I knew them, which was helpful for when the time came for me to get information from them. Anyway, this was a standing game that my dad played every Saturday morning, unless there was a University of Michigan home football game. Like every other Saturday, my father drove himself to the tennis facility. When he arrived to play, his tennis partners immediately noticed that there was something wrong with him. He seemed generally confused. What was most obvious was that he could not tie his tennis shoes.

From a discussion that I had with one of his tennis friends over the phone the day next day, I learned that my father was adamant about being okay and that he could drive himself home. He did not want to be taken to the hospital to be checked out. My father's tennis friends wanted to take him to the hospital but decided that because he was verbally refusing to go, they would drive him back home in his car and leave him with my mother, whose decision-making capabilities had been compromised due to her bike accident in 1985. To complicate matters, my mother had also had a mild stroke in 1996. I knew that she was drinking too much in the evenings and was no longer driving. Unfortunately, this "secret" was something that the guys from tennis did not know.

Two days had elapsed before my father was examined in an emergency room. The preliminary diagnosis was that he had suffered an Ischemic stroke. His stroke had probably occurred late Friday night or early Saturday morning. The amount of hours between the stroke and getting help interfered with the possibility of receiving crucial medical attention and treatment early on, which could have minimized the brain damage that he suffered.

At the time of my father's stroke, the use of a clot-busting drug like tPA (tissue Plasminogen Activator) may have been helpful in reducing the negative effects of the stroke. Had he been taken to the hospital upon recognition of his first symptoms perhaps the outcome would have been different. This we will never know.

I am writing about this, not as a medical doctor, making a medical recommendation, but to alert others of the importance of a quick response and treatment despite someone's resistance. Pick up the phone and call 911 if you have any suspicion that someone is having a stroke, or a heart attack.

When the response team arrives, they will handle the resistive individual with experience and with medical equipment and expertise to attend to the critical and time sensitive immediate needs of your family member. I do not blame his tennis buddies for the lack of appropriate action, because I understand that close friends have a difficult time going against someone's adamant refusal to do something.

My routine phone call home turned out to be a life-saving call. Those who dropped my dad off with my mom, figured she was capable of driving my father to the hospital or calling someone for help. There wasn't any further follow up from anyone. It was by happenstance that I found out what had happened. Things would have been much worse had I not been checking in on them.

Earlier Warning Signs

On that fateful day in, October of 1999, it all seemed to happen suddenly, but in reality it had been brewing for a long time. My father had been an attorney for fifty years. Approximately one year prior to his stroke, his law firm forced him into retirement. He was a very bright man, who was a "take charge" kind of personality, one might say controlling. At one level he recognized that his world was falling apart. He fought tooth and nail to hang onto his independence. His tenacity had been an asset in his younger, healthier days, but now it had become an impediment to recognizing the need to get help.

His health issues and onset of dementia had become a dangerous combination. Again, this type of situation can be found in many families. It is hard enough when your family in need lives nearby, but when you add the ingredient of long distance, with refusal on the part of the person to accept any outside assistance, the issues of need are critical and potentially traumatic, if not deadly.

During the summer months before my father's stroke in October, my sister came for her two or three week annual visit at the family cottage in Michigan. My husband and I also had a cottage next door. I was glad that she was there, not only to see her and spend time with her, but to get her take on my parents' declining health and ability to safely care for themselves. She quickly confirmed my concerns and noticed the same deterioration in my father's judgment and an increase in impulsivity and angry outbursts.

4

She often ran over to our cottage to get relief from being with my parents because it was hard to watch and hear and he was not rational about many things. His moods were quick to change and were unpredictable. We both felt that part of the problem was that his diabetic condition had become worse and his fluctuations in blood sugar might be part of the problem.

My father had been diagnosed with "brittle diabetes" and was managing his own injections. Brittle diabetes is a term used to describe hard-to-control swings in blood glucose levels. Not long before the tennis incident, he had gotten lost while driving and stopped at a gas station to figure out where he was and how to get home. Things were deteriorating and acceptance of any help on their part was out of the question. Yes, he went to the doctor, but he seemed to be able to cover up his confusion for short periods of time, such as a fifteen-minute office visit with his endocrinologist. I can imagine him shooting the breeze and making jokes and seeming just fine.

It was the day-to-day things that were not being handled as well by him as they had been in the past. This type of situation can be found in many families. For some odd reason, his A1C tests, a blood test that measures blood sugar spikes and averages, came back within the norm. In my father's case, this test was not picking up on the blood sugar swings and definitely could not detect the early signs of dementia, which became worse after his stroke.

We hoped that when our parents went back home at summer's end, that my father's endocrinologist would treat this change accordingly. With HIPPA laws and my father's irrationality, he was not open to our communication with his doctors at the time. We felt like we were between a rock and a hard place. In retrospect, today I would have picked up the phone and called his doctor and even if he could not give me any information, I could have told him what we were observing. The medical care that we could have gotten could have helped; however, we honestly were afraid of how he would react to us trying to get him to go in for a consultation. He had frequent episodes of hypoglycemia, which resulted in confusion, difficulty standing, sweating and shaking. He carried orange juice and candy with him wherever he went. He was still riding a bike and golfing, which burned calories. If he didn't dose himself properly with his insulin, or if he ate the wrong things, and didn't eat enough food, he did not do well.

We spent many hours trying to figure out the best way to intervene. For now, I vowed to keep a close eye on them; one of the blessings of having a place next door to them during the summer. I also knew that come September, I would be returning to Florida. One thing I was most worried about was his confusion during conversations, which was extremely unusual for him. One day, I was talking about something that had "flipped over" and he could not grasp what this meant and asked what in the world I was talking about. After taking an object and physically showing him what I was talking about, he got the concept. My mother looked at me with concern on her face and at this point I attributed the confusion to his blood sugar levels being so erratic, but I also wondered about possible TIA's (transient ischemic attacks), which is the term or acronym for "mini-strokes."

I went back home to Florida in September, and my parents returned to their home in Michigan. We were all terrified about their five hour drive home, but they miraculously made it safely. And, amazingly, my father attended his friends' son's graduation and my nephew's office party an hour and half away from home. I tried to convince them not to go but was already in Florida and could not stop them. Again, they made it some way, somehow, but it was not long thereafter the life-changing stroke that my father suffered occurred.

CHAPTER TWO

MY CAREGIVING JOURNEY FOR DAD BEGINS

I was on a plane the first thing the next morning after the call home on Halloween, and I remained in Michigan with my mother for five weeks until I could find another family member to "spell" me for a bit. While I stayed in Michigan, my husband "held down the fort" at home in Florida. Getting ready to leave was a flurry of activity and logistical arrangements. Thank God for my husband's support and help. It was very helpful to have someone who was not as emotionally wrapped up in what had happened, as I tried to organize things to leave at a moment's notice. The road that lay ahead was more difficult than I could have imagined. I truly had no clue what to expect and what I would find when I arrived in Michigan.

Seeing Dad in the Hospital—A Shock

Fortunately, my elderly aunt (my father's older sister), who lived an hour away from my parents, was able to go stay with my mother the first night that my father went to the hospital, the night before my arrival. I rented a car at the airport and drove directly to the hospital to be with my parents. The night before I arrived in Michigan, I had been told over the phone by the emergency room nurse, that my father would be admitted and that he had suffered a stroke but that he was oriented and alert. At that point, the extent of the damage done to his brain was not yet fully known. With the initial information that I had been given over the phone the night before, I thought that my father would be doing fairly well when I visited him in his room, but I was shocked to find that he was far worse than what I had expected.

In retrospect, I understand why the hospital staff was cautious about what they told me before I arrived, because I was travelling and they knew the risks involved in telling patients' family members too much before they arrive. It is standard practice of most hospitals to share only certain information over the phone. I also understand that I may have been in some denial about what I was facing, but a few things that I experienced when I first arrived at the Michigan hospital made things worse for me as a concerned family member.

Upon my arrival, the hospital was still in the process of evaluating his condition. The neurologist had not yet done his full work up, which turned out to be critical to our understanding how his abilities were impacted by his stroke. When I first appeared on the scene I did not fully understand what my dad had sustained and nobody was helping me to understand his condition, leaving me feeling panicked and powerless. How could I help him and my mother if nobody would talk to me and answer my questions? I did see a doctor writing notes outside my father's room.

I introduced myself and asked how my dad was doing. He barely looked up from his notes and said something like, "He's doing okay."

As I entered my father's room I recall having a feeling of hope, based upon what I had been told so far; however, what I saw did not match what I was being told by the medical staff at all. And, what I heard and felt was frightening to me. When I walked into my father's room he was in a bed by the window.

I said, "Hi Dad! It's Lin."

He never turned to look at me when he asked, "Where are you?"

I replied, "I just walked in the door of your room."

"I can't see you!" he said.

I walked over to his bed and touched him and said, "I'm right here Dad."

In front of him was a tray with food on a plate. He was not eating and I noticed that the right side of his plate did not have any food remaining; the food on the left side had obviously not been touched by him. I thought this was strange so I asked, "How's your meal? It looks like you hardly ate anything."

He shrugged his shoulders and said, "Not bad." I said, "You have quite a bit left on your plate."

He said, "No, I don't. I ate all of it."

I then realized that there was a distinct line between the foods that remained on the left side of his plate. I could only guess that he could not see the food on the left side of the plate or anything at all to the left of him, including me. I thought that my dad was blind and I could not figure out why not one person had told me this very important piece of information. I did not like what I was seeing. It did not jive with what I had been told by the Emergency Room staff or the nursing staff at the nursing station moments before I walked into his room. I fought back tears and told my dad that I would be right back.

I was filled with confusion, anger, fear and sadness. I remember my heart racing as I quickly exited the room to find someone to talk to about what was happening. The doctor I had just seen writing notes outside my dad's room assured me that my dad was not blind but that he had suffered a stroke that was affecting how he was processing sight. He did not explain why this was happening but told me the neurologist would be back to evaluate him either that evening or the next day. He emphasized that he was eating and able to walk and that he was able to speak. The doctor seemed nonplussed by my father's condition, which actually made me angry.

I remember feeling that the doctor and the staff were "going through the motions" and that they were not approachable. They seemed to be telling me things that did not accurately depict my father's condition. This would not be my last experience with this kind of communication from medical personnel in my fifteen-year journey. Of course, not all interactions were like this, nor as bad, but I can say that it didn't always go smoothly and part of the reason was because of my own state of mind at the time, but also because of the varying personalities of the health care personnel involved. The human factor can overshadow many situations and when emotions run high, this becomes more significant.

Thankfully, the neurologist came to examine my father that evening. He was personable, and connected well with my father as well as my mother and myself. My mother and I watched as the neurologist performed an assessment, which included talking to my father, and having him perform a few tasks involving speech, coordination and vision. He also asked my mother and me a few questions after he was finished with his basic exam. He or another neurologist had already done some preliminary tests upon arrival to the hospital, so he was there to see what improvements were already occurring, if any.

After I answered his questions, he then made a few comments that will always stick with me. "Your father is a very intelligent man. His stroke has caused something called "Left Neglect." The primary concerns with this condition is that a person's judgment is impaired and they are most often very impulsive; most importantly whatever is on the left side of him is not processed properly by the brain, which means he does not see anything on the left of him.

He explained that dad was not technically blind, his eye still worked fine, but what he should be seeing is not processed due to damage done by the stroke on the right side of the brain. My dad, because he had no significant speech impairment from the stroke, and he could walk without any problems, was at risk for getting places and not knowing where he was and making bad judgments about his personal affairs, such as issues having to do with money, safety, etc.

The neurologist went on to say that he would need therapeutic rehabilitation and from there we would be able to determine how much improvement and restoration of abilities would occur. Most significant to me was that the doctor strongly advised and warned that someone would need to take over all of his affairs. He explained that the primary issues of serious concern were that with "Left Neglect," comes impulsivity and poor judgment, meaning his safety was in jeopardy. I ended up being the person to "take over his affairs," as was advised. This was extremely overwhelming news for me to digest.

My questions of hope began with asking if my dad might ever drive again and the neurologist said that there was a possibility that he could regain this ability. This was something for my father to hang onto and strive for. To me, it didn't jive with what he had said about my father's limitations, but figured we'd cross that bridge when we got there.

The last thing the neurologist recommended was that my father be given more neuropsychological testing as soon as possible to assess his intellectual strengths and weakness. Along with this, physical, occupational, speech and language assessments were ordered and would begin immediately. He was to receive therapy while still in the hospital and then he would be reassessed once he was stabilized. It would then be determined by the team where he would go to live upon discharge from the hospital. At this point, we didn't know if this would mean he'd be sent home or somewhere else. In the meantime, I needed to get paperwork in place to take over my father and mother's affairs and I would stay at my parents' house to take care of my mom.

What I learned and understood more about later was that there was a chance that the left neglect could reverse with time and therapy. This gave us some hope to hang onto in the beginning; however, despite this feeling of hope, I was devastated and did not feel optimistic at all. I could not believe what I was being told. I was besieged by worries, "What will we do if...? Will he get better? Is the brain damage permanent? Can therapy "fix" the problem? What about my mom? How long will I need to stay in Michigan? How do I find the right place for him to receive therapy?" On the flip side, I also remember not wanting to know what lay ahead. I wished that time would stand still, or that I could get back on the plane and return home. On top of this, I was exhausted and emotionally raw. I remember feeling conflicted and uncertain about my options.

My Reactions

Whenever I questioned or considered my choices, even just to myself, it made me feel like a bad daughter. I remember wondering if there was any way possible for me to extricate myself from this situation. Then I felt ashamed that I could even think this way, as my parents' lives were literally on the line. This type of thinking and feeling isn't unusual at all. Unfortunately, when I or others are faced with being ripped away from our own lives and families, even temporarily, it is only normal to have feelings of selfishness, anger and deep sadness for the changes we imagine are ahead of us, or right in front of us.

For me personally, I was in the middle of a two-year leave of absence from my school social work position in Michigan and was embarking on a new direction in my own career/life. My first children's book for traumatized and grieving children had been published the year before, and I was actively consulting and talking to schools and other mental health professional groups in South Florida. I was enjoying my freedom and knew that things were going to change for me quickly. The most significant feeling I recall having was one of panic, rooted in the sense that I had to button up my life, without really knowing what lay ahead for my family and myself. I was scared but knew that I needed to remain in control in order to be helpful. My life was suddenly on hold.

This selfish feeling is not unusual and it affects most people when they are first faced with dropping their lives to take care of someone else at a moment's notice. What is important to recognize though is that the feelings are normal and should not be ignored or held inside. How each individual copes may be different and this can be attributed to a variety of factors, which I will discuss later on in the book. Taking care of oneself is essential to being able to truly help someone else effectively. This is not a new concept, but honestly it cannot be said enough to those of us who are in the role of caregiver.

Organizing Someone Else's Life

It would be nice if the people we have stepped in to help lived in an organized way so that we could easily find important documents, papers, etc. In my case, my elderly parents did not have things so that I could find what I needed in an easy way. This could probably be prevented with pre-planning, which again was something my family refused to do.

Believe it or not, and I could not believe it, my parents had only recently drawn up a Will, which was the result of a dinner that my husband and I had with my parents where my mother said to us, "Can you believe your lawyer father doesn't have a Will?" Here was my father, a lawyer, and he did not have a Will. This was based upon his entrenched denial and unrecognized dementia, which we did not know about, except for the occasional irrational outbursts of anger and recent low blood sugar episodes which effected his orientation, for example getting lost driving in his home town.

At the time of my father's stroke there were no Advanced Health Care Directives. Control, or the fear of a loss of control was overriding my father's ability to make some important decisions in his life. Come to find out, he wasn't the only one of my aging relatives who was operating this way, which I would learn later about my aunt and uncle and my brother as well, even though these options were available to them.

Taking Care of Mom: Our History Didn't Help

While my father remained in the hospital and began his therapy and built up his strength, I took care of my mother in their home. It was an experience to remember. I loved my mother, but she and I had very different temperaments. This was true since I was a young child. I remember my mom telling me that I would not take a nap like my brother and sister had.

I was high energy and busy, which was difficult for her after having been diagnosed with Polio shortly after I was born. She was sent to the hospital and remained there in an "Iron Lung" ward during much of my first six months of my life. In addition to Polio, she told me later in life that she also had encephalitis. This early separation and disruption to our family effected all of us and in differing ways.

I mention this aspect of my mother's life, because it made a difference for our mother/daughter relationship with respect to our sense of closeness. I loved my mother, and we had some things in common that we loved to talk about, like horses and animals, and this seemed to be our most significant bond. But before I started Kindergarten at age five, I do not remember playing games with her. I do remember her sleeping a lot, which was related to her illness.

Because of our different personalities and our early bonding interruption, we had love but not the affectionate bond that many mothers and daughters have. My sister told me that my mother actually talked about the fact that she felt that she had not bonded with me as she had with my brother and her, because she could not hold or take care of me for quite some time after I was born. Within three or four weeks of my mother giving birth to me, she was whisked away from me and put into quarantine. They reportedly would hold me up to a window in the door, so my mom could see her baby, me.

My brother and sister were sent to grandparents, and I had a nurse nanny during the day when my father was at work. He then took over in the evenings and took care of me himself. Stories told about the "nurse" who cared for me were that when my father was late coming home, and when it got dark outside, she would hide in a closet out of fear, because our house was in a wooded area.

Stories like this stuck with me and explained some of why I had the feelings about my mom that I did. It also explained my feeling closer to my father even though I was jealous of my brother who got most of my father's attention. Ironically, I ended up being the one who took care of my parents due to proximity and availability later in life. This is important, because I feel that the opportunity to be with my mother and my father in their times of need helped to heal old wounds and built a closeness that we never really had shared at a deeper level.

It is also important to reiterate, that my mother had experienced a serious bike accident in 1985, resulting in a closed head injury, which happened on the eve of my thirtieth birthday, and right before my new job as a school social worker was to start one week later. This accident was traumatic for our family. At that point in time, my father was still very capable of taking care of my mother. She was hospitalized for approximately five weeks and my father was her primary caregiver. I had my own life, was married and I was living about one hour from them. My father's life certainly changed significantly after my mother's head injury. I honestly believe that the stress of being a caregiver for my mother may have accelerated and exacerbated his own health issues.

Without going into the details of this accident, the most significant part of this life event for all of us, was that my mother was never the same after it happened. She was not as quick mentally, her affect or facial expressions were no longer as expressive, she had a poor short- term memory and she was even slower in everything that she did than before the accident. The reason behind this accident affected my feelings toward my mother in a negative way, because she had contributed to it happening, as she was biking under the influence of alcohol. I feel guilty about sharing this information as I type it, but I also know that I am not alone in having a family with issues of alcohol and/or substance abuse. With such concerns, accidents caused by overindulging, may complicate how we feel about the incident.

I loved my mother and understood that she had a problem with drinking too much at the time of her accident. This factor affected my feelings significantly. I understood things from an intellectual perspective based upon my professional training and background, yet emotionally I had a hard time not feeling angry at her for hurting herself, because of what I saw was her fault. I also was angry with my father, for not taking care of her as I thought he should.

Fortunately, I had gone to a therapist during the beginning of my professional social work career, which I felt was essential to my ability to help others. I had ended therapy before the accident happened but was able to contact him to return to counseling when this family crisis occurred. Therapy helped me to sort through my own feelings toward my parents, which ultimately helped me cope better with my relationship with both of my parents. Acceptance of what I could and could not control was big for

14

me. The point of my sharing this is to point out the importance of finding someone whom you can trust to talk to when you are having difficulty with coping with family issues and relationships, especially when a crisis occurs. For me, it made all the difference.

So, I came into the "call" to help my mother with a lot of baggage, years of unresolved anger and frustration toward her. Despite this, we managed to come together on behalf of my father and we did quite well. In retrospect, due to the fact that I was not as close to my mother as I always felt my sister was, I was able to see things, I think, more realistically sometimes. I could see the way things were for my mother and my father and I didn't have a rose-colored perception of things. This helped when I made the decision to step in and help. I think the fact that I wasn't enmeshed in their situation made it easier for me to look at what lay ahead and what had to be done. I quickly got past the idea that they could stay at home and live happily ever after. I knew that things had to change and it needed to happen sooner rather than later.

Back To Dad

Before the stroke, both of my parents were very resistant to even considering moving and any attempt by family to look into getting them some help was met with rage on my father's part. He managed to intimidate everyone who cared about him to keep the subject of moving or getting extra help at bay. Denial was a common defense mechanism in our family system, so not planning for the future played right into the hand of keeping our heads deeply embedded in the sand. Yes, we talked about ways to encourage mom and dad to accept the help that they needed, and, yes, we thought they should move out of their home, but my parents' adamant resistance kept me at bay, so no help was given or arranged.

These were my parents, who were adults, who could not be forced to do anything that they didn't agree to doing. My parents were not close to any current neighbors, and their best friends had moved away or had problems of their own. Before the stroke we worried about dad driving and even suggested to him that he should not drive. Of course I can hear him yelling back that that would never happen. I did not realize how bad his driving was until I took my mother to see him in the hospital after his stroke.

The first time I drove her to see to see him, she began shouting out driving instructions, such as, Stop, Green, Red, whenever we approached a Stop sign or traffic light. It unnerved me and made me jump the first few times it occurred. I said to my mother, "Why are you yelling these instructions at me while I'm driving? Is that what you had to do when you drove with Dad?"

She answered, "Yes!" Oh my God, I thought. How scary is that?

So I said, "Wow, it must have been really scary to drive with him." She admitted that it was.

I then assured her that I could see the lights and stop signs, so she didn't have to be my eyes, like she was for Dad. My father's diabetes had caused a condition called retinopathy, which causes blindness without treatment. He was receiving treatment, and was not yet legally blind however, his eyesight was not good and he should not have been driving. I still shudder when I think of how lucky they were not to have or caused a major traffic accident and harmed or killed someone else or themselves. That was a miracle. This is where I take issue with the fact that driver licenses for the elderly are renewed without testing, which I think is very dangerous. This issue came up with every one of the elderly family members that I cared for. Bottom line, it took a major life crisis for things to change.

Coping with Changes

It was time to move forward and do what was best for my parents, which meant figuring out so many things; things I had never had to do before. Uncharted territory is scary for anyone, and I was definitely scared. We had time to work on a move, but not a lot of time. So many decisions had to be made and so much needed to be done. My head was spinning.

My father had been released to Skilled Nursing care from the hospital and was receiving physical, occupational and speech and language therapy. The facility was not far from their home; the house I lived in from the time I was born, until I got married. I was fortunately very familiar with the community, which was a huge benefit to my making my way around town. This may not be the case for many people. I ended up staying with my mother for five straight weeks to get things in order. I was hesitant to ask for anyone to give me time to go home. I felt that it was my duty and responsibility to stay and help my mother and to monitor my father's care, which was fine, but it affected my entire life.

It took time to know the degree of cognitive ability, physical strength and self-care skills my father would regain. Unfortunately, not even the experts could predict how much self-sufficiency my father would regain; nor did they want to discourage him or the family. They could not tell us exactly how long he would be there or how much progress he would make. All of this information would have been very helpful in our decision-making process. I think that the tendency to cushion someone's prognosis is done with good intentions and with sensitivity to the patient and family members; however, when you are feeling pressed for time to figure out what to do, it can feel very frustrating. So, the roller-coaster ride began, and it was not a fun ride!

CHAPTER THREE

CARE PLANNING, MOVES, REACHING OUT, MAKING DECISIONS

My father initially received physical, speech and language and occupational therapy while in the hospital. I am not sure of the exact timeline, but after stabilizing him medically, and developing a treatment plan with goals, it was recommended by the Michigan hospital team of professionals, along with the medical social worker, that my father be moved to a skilled nursing facility. In other words, he would live in the facility in a therapeutic milieu, where all of his care, including medical, physical and therapeutic needs would be met. My mother would stay at home and I would stay there with her until we knew more.

Opposition

The first move for my father was from the hospital to the Skilled Nursing facility near their home. Seemed like a great choice to me but not to my dad. In his mind, he was fine and well enough to go straight home from the hospital. This is not an unusual response for most people who are elderly, especially with dementia and issues of poor judgment.

The professional recommendation to go somewhere other than home was met with much resistance. My experience working with oppositional and defiant children as a social worker came in handy with my father throughout my caregiving experience with him. This was the beginning of many rough transitions. He was not always easy to deal with before the stroke, but now his behavior was impacted by his cognitive condition, poor judgment and I am sure underlying fear. I knew it wasn't going to be easy, but I also knew I had to be the one to support the process. This was the first of several moves for my father.

I took advantage of going on a tour of the facility, which was suggested and arranged by the hospital social worker. I learned prior to my visit, that my father would receive more therapy, within a setting that could also provide medical management. His diabetes was difficult to control and he was not able to give himself his own shots anymore due to his stroke. The skilled nursing center was designed to provide the therapeutic milieu for him to learn the daily living skills necessary to adapt to his new deficits caused by the stroke.

Helping him to learn how to eat or more specifically, feed himself, walk safely, and accept assistance from others were primary goals established by the therapy staff. At this point, I was learning myself along the way about things like the differences between assisted living and skilled nursing facilities, which I will explain later.

Opting For the Less Desirable

I was included in all meetings, because my father's judgment had been impaired by the stroke as well. My mother was in no position to manage her life, let alone these meetings. My aunt and uncle, who at this time were still functioning fairly well independently, came almost daily to visit my father. This kind of family support was a Godsend, not just for my father, but for me, too. Finding the right place for my dad was not easy. Essentially, I had to settle on what was available, not necessarily the optimal placement, because the better of the two skilled nursing facilities in the area was full, so we had to opt for the less desirable skilled nursing center.

The building was very nice, but their staffing was not good and the care was sometimes substandard in my assessment. I felt very uncomfortable leaving my father there alone and felt very guilty every time I left to go back home to Florida. The positive point about this facility was that they were able to house my mother for "respite care" when no family member could be in town to stay with her in her home. This was an excellent option for a few reasons. It was a good way to have my mother's capabilities assessed based upon the nursing staff's observations and feedback. She had supervision while no family or friends could stay with her. The house was riddled with problems that had been ignored for years and needed fixing, such has holes in the ceilings.

Planning the Next Move

While my father was in Skilled Nursing care and receiving therapy, I began to explore where my parents could move when the time came. I listened to input from the professionals, word of mouth, and the Internet as a starting point. The top choices at the time were either to move into a facility in Michigan, stay at home with outside help coming in, stay in long term care where he was being treated at the time, or move in with a family member, and lastly, near my husband and me in Florida. The choices in Michigan at the time were limited. After researching and visiting what was available in the area where they lived, the consensus was to sell their home as soon as my father could handle the rigors of moving. What I do recall is that one of the first things I needed to do was to understand the differences between what Assisted Living was and had to offer, and the same for Skilled Nursing Care and Long Term Care. It was all new to me at this point.

In 1999, I honestly did not know what Assisted Living was. Today, it is a common term and there are far more facilities for assisted living. Now, many people know what this type of care facility is, or at the very least has heard the term through advertisement or friends whose family is living in one. However, many still do not fully understand what such a place has to offer. One thing I found out quickly is that all Assisted Living places are not created equally, or managed, staffed or run the same. Research had to be done to figure out what would be the best fit for my parents based upon what the medical, rehabilitation and psychological evaluations recommended. The neurologist maintained some optimism for my father, as did the neuro-psychologist and the physical therapy team, but also warned of my father's limitations.

Care Planning

I made a point of being at every Care Planning meeting on behalf of my father. The patient can be a participant in such meetings; however, for my father, it was suggested that he not attend, so I acted as my father's representative at every meeting. My father did not need any added stress and was not in a position to make decisions based upon his mental status from the stroke. I agreed with this recommendation. I was able to represent my father and mother, because I had done the proper legal paperwork and permission assigning me as his Patient Advocate. In Florida the same assignment is called a Health Care Surrogate. I agreed with this recommendation. We also felt that my mother need not be in attendance either although I do remember occasions when she did come, so that she had a better understanding of my father's condition and care.

Care planning meetings include the professionals providing therapeutic rehabilitation. My father's meetings included a social worker, speech and language, physical and occupational therapist and nutritionist in attendance and each would give a report.

They reviewed and reported everything from what my father's weight was to how he participated or did not participate in activities. Speech and language concerns, coordination and social and emotional status were discussed. The participants also noted whether or not he appeared depressed, confused or anxious. All reports gauged his overall status, improvement, decline or regression.

My background came in very handy in the Care Planning meetings, in that I had worked with such treatment teams in my own work and I knew what questions to ask and could follow the terminology. My questions were typically in response to what was reported. It is important to listen carefully to each report, and if you don't understand what they are saying, or want more information, you can and should be able to ask questions at any point during the meeting. For example, if they said my father was not cooperating, eating or being disruptive, I asked for specific examples, simply by saying, how is my dad not cooperating, or does he eat better at different times of day? Specific questions in response to what is being reported is the key to getting the best plans in place to address the physical, social and medical concerns in a constructive way. Discussion should be a part of the care plan meetings. I did find that some meetings were more productive and professional than others over my course of caregiving. Just like individual personalities, each system has their own approach and way of doing things. I recall some meetings where the staff seemed rushed and as if they were giving an impersonal report on anyone in the facility. I also had experiences that showed that my family member was known well and not just another face in the crowd.

I should say that if you have questions from concerns regarding care or treatment, bring them up during the meeting. Come prepared! Write down your questions ahead of the meetings, because it is very easy to forget once you're in a meeting. These meetings can be stressful, and under stress we often lose our train of thought or go blank and can't think of what to ask, or we might feel intimidated and shy. It is also okay to bring someone with you if you would like, and if possible, you should let the staff contact person or meeting coordinator, who most oftentimes is the social worker, know ahead of time. All of this is okay and to be expected.

The patient can be a participant in such meetings; however, for my father, it was suggested that he not attend, so I acted as my father's representative at every meeting. My father did not need any added stress and was not in a position to make decisions based upon his mental status from the stroke. I agreed with this recommendation. We also felt that my mother need not be in attendance either although I do remember occasions when she did come, so that she had a better understanding of my father's condition and care.

An additional issue was that when I was back in Florida and I could not physically be in attendance, a conference call was done instead so that I could participate in the meeting. From these meetings, I was able to get a better handle on what I needed to do next for my parents.

Taking A Break, Asking for Help: Not So Easy

One of the other things that I needed to do was have someone come in and give me a chance to go home, regroup, look into options for my parents where I lived. It had been five weeks away from home and I needed to figure out a way to leave my mother and father and get some respite and time to put my life in order and prepare for moving my parents. This was not an easy decision, nor was it easy to do. Leaving my mother was not easy, but it was the right thing to do.

As it turned out, I reached out to my sister after my first five weeks living with my mother in Michigan. The thing that made it more difficult for me to ask her for help, or to spell me, was that in January of 1997, my sister's forty-eight year old husband of twenty-five years had died in a plane crash. This was a tragic event for our entire family. Her two sons were both in college at the time of my brother-in-law's death. This was another layer added onto my parents' situation. My sister, who had been a pre-school owner and teacher, had just started a Master of Divinity program in Denver, Colorado. So, she was also far away from my parents and had a lot on her plate already, including a very recent major move out of the town she lived in for approximately twenty years raising her family in Wyoming.

I knew my sister was coping with her own grief and issues of a major life change, but I needed to go home for a bit, and I was feeling distraught and exhausted and had nowhere else to turn but to my sister. I felt guilty for bothering her, but also knew I needed to get back home to my husband and responsibilities in Florida. My sister had to figure out her own timeline and availability. Thanks to her willingness and to a Christmas break from her schooling for the holidays, she flew to Michigan so I could orient her and "show her the ropes." She stayed through Christmas and I returned shortly afterward, overlapping with her for the handoff of responsibilities.

I found for myself that one of the most difficult things for me to do was to ask for help. I was lucky in that I did have family who was able to provide some respite from time to time, but within the process of asking for help came lots of feelings and issues. Specifically, when we are the designated "helper," it can create many feelings and logistical issues whenever we must leave to take care of our own lives. Everyone deals with the dilemma of leaving differently. However, I contend that most people feel guilty as they leave someone behind who is facing a major health concern, life changes and an inability to express their wants and needs. I was an advocate for my family members, which meant I was oftentimes their voice and connection to those who could help them. As I walked out the door, I felt that I was abandoning them and it was not a good feeling at all.

To add to this, oftentimes when I would take a break, it felt and was actually more difficult than staying "on duty" and doing it all myself. And, being a controlling person, I had difficulty giving up the reins to someone else. I figured that they would be temporary and knew I was in it for the long haul. I will cover this dilemma further as each caregiving experience presented this same recurring issue, but with added differences and concerns. I wish I could say that it got easier every time, but honestly for me it didn't. I did learn that I needed to step aside and accept help and I was better able to take the breaks I needed, but I never felt good about leaving and worried the entire time I was away.

The Problems with Making a Decision

While back in Florida, my husband and I began looking into different levels of care facilities for my parents, if and/or when we might decide to move them to Florida near us. My sister took over in Michigan and followed up on the two places recommended to me by the Michigan therapy team. Back then, the choices were few in Michigan, whereas Florida could provide many more and better options for much less cost. As with anything, this discrepancy in supply and cost was based in the principle of "supply and demand." As one person on one of my flights told me, "Florida is God's waiting room." That stuck with me and to be honest there is much truth to this.

Conflicting Signs of Progress

My mother continued to need support, as did my father. Plans were on hold, while tentative plans were being made with respect to where they might live when my father was well enough to leave the skilled nursing center/assisted living home. I know this doesn't sound like it makes sense, but that's the way it was because the doctors and therapists could not predict how far my father's healing would go.

The term "plateau" is used to mark a time in treatment or therapy, where a person stops making progress in their capabilities. An easy example is that someone may not be able to speak at all immediately after a stroke, or they may not be able to use their right hand. Treatment goals are established and periodic reviews are done to see how much function is regained in speech or mobility. Occupational, speech and language and physical therapists would most often be those providing the therapy and would provide the progress reports.

In my father's case, he did show some early improvement in speech and mobility, but his left neglect, judgment and self-care skills reached a point where no more progress was being made. This was significant to our plans for my father. What was good in his case was that therapy would be offered again when he moved into a more permanent residence or facility. And, therapy can be reinstituted if skills decline after a six week period of time, while living in care facilities.

Finances

After my sister spelled me for about two weeks, I had to fly back to Michigan to again stay with my mother and go for daily visits with my father, meet with those who were caring for him and attend care conferences which reminded me of my meetings for students and clients when I was a social worker. This part of secondary caregiving actually felt most comfortable to me.

On the other hand an aspect of caregiving that was difficult for me was dealing with the banks and the accountants. While with my mother, one of my essential tasks was for me to try to pay bills, which called for making sense of my parents' check ledgers, which had clearly deteriorated greatly in terms of organization and legibility in recent months. My father's handwriting had changed and his math didn't add up. I am no mathematician, however, that was one of my father's strengths. My mother always told me, "I hate math," which I emulated growing up. In fact, I vividly recalled my parents having big fights when I was growing up over my mom's mistakes in the checkbook. After her head injury, my father took over everything, so I knew that she was not able to help me.

Trying to piece together my parents' life was like doing a jigsaw puzzle, without all of the pieces available to me. I spent hours making phone calls and looking through records to see what I could do to get payments made, etc. It didn't take me long to figure out that not only did I need to take over my father's affairs, just like the neurologist had said, but it was clear that someone should have stepped in much sooner. My father must have been so stressed, on top of being in denial that he needed help. I was now the one feeling extremely stressed and overwhelmed, with a feeling of where do I start?

For now, just understand that my father's financial picture was not good and what was needed for his care was going to be expensive. This is where pre-planning is so important. I'm no Suzi Orman, the TV financial expert, but I can tell you that when financial planning is not done properly, when medical crises strike or aging issues take over, things are that much more difficult without a plan. As I took over all of the bill paying I began to understand that my parents' world had already been unraveling for quite some time.

I hope by hearing my issues that it will save you some time and give you some comfort to understand that when you take over someone else's life it can feel like drowning in a sea of paperwork, and that you are not alone in this type of situation. It takes time and patience to get everything in order and figured out. And, for me it was very difficult to have this responsibility hanging over my head. When I was lost, I knew enough to ask questions, no matter how dumb they seemed to me.

My brother could not figure out just how in the world my father, after being a successful attorney for fifty years, had so little money. He questioned me, in what felt like a challenging way, in his amazement over how bad our parents' financial situation was. He really seemed to have no idea that my parents' lives were in complete upheaval on every level. I felt defensive when questioned by my siblings and resented being doubted when I told of the reality of my parents' situation.

The bottom line was that they could not live independently anymore with the information that I had at this point, based upon the professionals treating my father and their financial status. For all of us, the reality of the circumstances that my parents were in was not easy for us to face or accept! The wish was that they could stay in their home. Realistically this was not the best choice.

Fear of Making the Wrong Choice

Change under the best case scenario can be difficult, but add all the ingredients that were in my father's situation and it is challenging to say the least. I found myself doubting and questioning decisions and recommendations due to my own difficulty with looking at the reality of the changes ahead for my parents. It is sad, scary and life altering when such changes are necessary and we're not ready for them. Intellectually I totally understood and agreed with what was being recommended, but when the actual transition from the skilled nursing facility to the assisted living center was suggested, I felt remorse and sorrow. This, I knew, was the beginning of the end of my parents' independent living and their lives and logically I understood these steps of change were necessary; however, I was more than fearful of making the wrong choices.

As an aside, my husband told me from the beginning that I would need a Power of Attorney to take over my father's affairs. I was fortunate in that I was able to reach out to my father's law firm where he last worked for help. And, yes, I was very lucky to have this option. I could go to someone whom I trusted, but most importantly, someone my father knew and trusted for help. If you do not have a family attorney, I would suggest asking friends of someone they used or knew, or Googling elder care attorneys. For my first experience with getting the proper paperwork in order, I was lucky enough to know someone. The main thing to remember is not to try to figure this all out alone. My husband and I had already gotten such things in place for ourselves in our thirties, so the fact that my parents did not have anything, except a newly drafted will, was surprising.

Not Realizing the Extent of Dad's Dementia

I think what I regret most is that none of us knew the extent of my father's dementia, which had clearly started before his retirement. My husband recognized a problem, dating back to when his own father died in 1988, and my father handled the estate for my husband. My father, after five years, had not closed the estate. He had all of the information that he needed, but he just couldn't seem to pull it altogether to complete the process. Finally, one day my husband said to me, "You have to intercede. This has gone on far too long. It seems like your dad is prolonging this, either because he is incompetent, or he's doing it on purpose. Please say something to him. I need to put this behind me and it is very upsetting to me. If I bring it up to your father, I am afraid of what I might say." he said. This was a huge red flag!! My husband saw it all more clearly and objectively. I didn't want to recognize that my father was slipping mentally; because of his intelligence, he covered his deficits well.

Confirmation of what we suspected but didn't act upon, was verified when I needed to call upon my father's prior secretary, whom I asked to come help us with some files that he had stored in the garage of their home. There were stacks and stacks of old case files in boxes. We had encouraged my father to do some legal work from home, after he was asked to leave the last law firm for which he was not a partner, as he had been in previous firms, but was considered to be "Of Counsel."

Our own denial, and the lack of information given to us by the law firm regarding my father's difficulty with completing things, led us to encourage my father to do something which we never should have done. What I found out from his former secretary, was that my father was not able to finish things and was having difficulty with organization. Her comments brought me back to a time when my mother started to tell us about a situation my father was having with a client involving him being sued for an error and omission. My father would not let her go on any further, so we never found out what this all meant.

Later I came to understand that he had what is termed deficits in "executive cognitive functioning." He could talk about doing things, think about doing things, but he could not act on his thoughts and ideas nor complete things. This is usually due to frontal lobe damage in the brain. The secretary sharing her own experience with my father's decline shed new light on what we all suspected. What I now know is that she covered for my father's limitations and deficits and she watched as he became less and less capable to practice law. This explained the request by the firm that he retire. And, this was against his wishes.

Sadly, that summer he lashed out at me right away when my husband and I went to help him and my mother carry luggage to the cottage upon their arrival. He snapped at me, "You know I can ostracize people who treat me like I'm old." I recall thinking, that's a weird thing to say. Where did that come from? Later on, when everything came to a head for my father, things all came together for me.

My father was devastated by his "retirement" and never even shared that it had happened with any of the family. He was ashamed. He was seventy-seven, I believe, when it all came down. Dementia had trumped his intelligence and ability to cover up his problems. His own father prided himself on hanging onto his business until he was seventy-nine. He wanted to work forever; it was his world, it was his identity. Being asked to leave was a crushing blow to his ego. This is why, when we realized this, my husband and I, not knowing the extent of his problems, encouraged him to take on cases independently, mostly for friends. This didn't last long.

I share this background to show readers that even with my social work experience and diagnostic skills, when it came to my father, I did not want to see what was happening. Denial kept me from seeing the truth. I could not look at the obvious decline in my father's capabilities head on. As I explained in the early part of my father's story, he was not receptive to help, so I have forgiven myself for my lack of direct intervention and action. Perhaps it could have made a difference, but what I did was the only thing that I knew and thought was best at the time.

Moving Both Parents from Their Home

After my father's stroke, coupled with my mother's inability to manage life solo, and the need for medical assistance and safety concerns, as well as financial concerns, it was apparent that with these ingredients, the best answer for my parents was for them to move out of their home and into a care facility.

For me, the thought of moving my parents seemed to be a monumental task. First, they did not want to move. Second, their house was in need of work and would be a "tear down," but it also needed repairs to prepare it for a sale. On top of things like roof leaks their home hadn't been cleaned in some time. It just so happened that a tree had crashed through a large plate glass window one of the first nights I stayed with my mother due to a bad storm. This had to be fixed as soon as possible. Fortunately, I knew the name of the handy man/builder whom my parents had used through the years and befriended. I was able to call him and ask for his help, which saved some money and time.

More Opposition

Another part of preparation for sale was to help my mother come to a place of acceptance of the idea. Her resistance to moving was of course based upon emotion not logic, which I understood, but I wasn't sure how to deal with in the beginning. After giving it much thought, I opted to not tell her that she would definitely be moving, but instead to tell her that we need to keep the option of selling their home, in case this was what was recommended by the people caring for dad. I added that we would ask the doctors and therapists what they thought would be best for dad.

Using the doctors and professionals as the people who could guide us along the way, helped take me out as the mean daughter who was the one suggesting that they be taken away from the life they had known, as well the place they had called home for most of their adult lives. Big changes had already come and more would be coming, which for my mother, for anyone, was a lot to take in all at once on so many levels. Her resistance was normal, but what added to the difficulties were her cognitive and memory limitations.

I needed to be aware of what to share and how to share information while trying to remain sensitive to what she was facing and going through. Was this easy? No, it was not. What we know intellectually, does not always match how we process things emotionally. I found myself in a constant state of ambivalence, which led to self-doubt at the same time. I felt very conflicted around how to make it all happen and needed someone to support my decisions. Add to this an element of grief over losing the parents who were strong, capable individuals.

Uncertainty

This feeling of uncertainty was something that ran through all of my caregiving experiences, but with my parents, I think it was the worst. I attribute this to the shift of roles that happens when we as "children" move into the one making the decisions. Obviously, this can be overcome, but it warrants mentioning and recognizing, because this shift impacts how we as caregivers cope with the changes. So the thought of moving my parents seemed to me to be a monumental task. I felt pressured and a bit like a fish out of water, but had to forge ahead, be strong and make sure that I stayed connected with those taking care of my parents whether I was in Florida, or in Michigan.

I learned a lot about logistics as a result. I was completely overwhelmed by what it would take to get them out of their home. My solution was to approach this task by asking questions, making lists and figuring out who I needed to help me. It meant selling the house, which meant moving forty-five years of life long possessions, memories and just plain old stuff that was never thrown away.

As the idea of moving was on the table, I continued to deal with the day-to-day tasks at hand—visits to see my father every day, while taking care of all my parents' business affairs, paying bills, making appointments with lawyers, visiting banks and sifting through paperwork to try to make sense of their lives.

I needed to weigh the professionals' advice, along with what we as a family could handle, arrange and live with, coupled with consideration of my parents' feelings. Once the decisions were in place, then the nitty-gritty of organizing rears its ugly head. I can still remember the feeling of thinking, "where do I begin?"

It was essential that I talk to people, because what I found is that sometimes someone has gone through a similar experience, not the same mind you, but some piece of our situation, so they may have some useful advice or suggestions. Case in point. A very good friend in Florida, whose parents had recently moved to Florida, gave me the name of a business near my parents' place that would do an estate sale for us, prior to putting the house on the market. He told me who to call, and what to expect, which took a load off of my mind. At the same time, I needed to find someone to help pull everything together for an estate sale.

31

Finding a Balance

From the point of my father's stroke at the end of October of 1999, to the time that we moved him and my mother in the beginning of February 2000, was only three months; however, it seemed like an eternity to me.

This distortion of time appeared in each one of my caregiving experiences. I know this was a distortion of perception, and I believe it was rooted in my feelings of loss and sadness, along with feeling ripped away from my home. I'm a bit of a homebody, not interested in taking long trips, so every time I had to leave I dreaded it. This sounds selfish, I know, but it's honestly how I felt and I am sure others also feel this way. Yes, I coped with it and pulled myself up by my bootstraps and did what had to be done. These feelings were constantly coming at me as part of the process of long distance caregiving. To top it off, then when I would get back home, I felt guilty for leaving my husband behind; a true "catch 22."

I know that I flew back and forth several times from Florida to Michigan, but cannot tell you how many times; it seemed like too many. My focus was to stay on top of my father's care, look out for my mother's needs, prepare for a potential move for my parents, and research what would be best for my parents while tending to my own life. It was a matter of juggling my life and theirs, trying to attend to each while not ignoring the other. My own life was taking a backseat at this point in the family crisis. This is not unusual and to be expected. The fact that this is not unusual doesn't mean that it is easy.

My transition, from my parents' "world" to my own home life, was challenging. I was distracted and exhausted both emotionally and physically and wanted to talk with someone about what happened with my father, mother, the plans I had to make, and the stress I was under. But at the same time, I didn't want to burden my husband with my issues and spend all of our time together rehashing what I had been through in Michigan. This doesn't mean he wouldn't help me or listen to me, because he did. However, there were times of awkwardness and times he didn't want to hear the blow-by-blow of my time away. He wanted my attention to be on our life.

I found it difficult to find a balance, and was trying to please everyone all the time. This is not an uncommon trend for caregivers, but it is something we need to attend to. Trying to be the "hero" and handle everything ourselves takes its toll. And, my underlying anger toward my parents' situation didn't help.

What I resented most was the fact that my parents had resisted help before things came to a head, and that was what was overshadowing my acceptance or anger about the situation in which I found myself. This was something I had to reckon with in each caregiving experience I had, but this first "trial by fire" was very distressing from the get go. So I would have the occasional personal "pity party" and move on to what had to be done for my parents and figure out a way to find the energy for my husband after my difficult trips home and back.

At this point in my caregiving role, I did not realize that I needed someone to talk to who was neutral, not a family member. This was ironic, considering my profession as a helper that I didn't reach out for help. To be honest, I couldn't figure out when I would have time to do this anyway, so I trudged along and would find myself complaining to friends and family and realized people didn't want to listen. I needed to figure out some other ways to release my stress.

It took time for me to find ways to take care of me. Finding a balance is one goal to try to maintain, but of course this is often easier said than done. Setting small goals worked for me. Setting lofty goals did not always work. For example, a small goal might be taking a fifteen-minute bath, where I could shut the door and breathe and remove myself from responsibility and thinking about what I must do next. This can be very relaxing and greatly rejuvenating. Small self-gifts like this can be very helpful.

The bottom line is that I was faced with lots of firsts in my maiden caregiving role for sure, and I am sure this is true for many people who end up being in this position through necessity. Add to this, the uncertainty that life holds anyway and you will undoubtedly feel stressed. One aspect that always added to my feelings was the long distance factor. I faced continuous time constraints and a balancing act between my life, travel, my parents' lives and figuring out how to fit everything in. I remember thinking about how if only I lived down the street, things would be easier; not stress free, just filled with fewer logistics and the overshadowing feeling of urgency. The need for balance was something that would frequently come up for me with taking care of my parents' lives. I felt torn and stressed by my newfound role and at first was not sure how to handle the pushing, pulling and tugging in so many different directions.

CHAPTER FOUR

PAST ANY HOPE OF GOING HOME

During my sister's visit home around Christmas time, while my father was in the Assisted Living, he was still anxious to go "home." My sister and I both thought it would be a good idea to take him for a visit to see how he managed the experience. My father's therapists and doctors agreed we should try it. We all thought that it would be very telling as to whether or not the idea of them moving home with home care assistance was truly an option or not. Plus, it would be good for his mental health to have an outing.

We had been doing some lunch and dinner outings to some of his favorite area restaurants so it was time to test how he handled a trip home; a place that would be most familiar to him. The home visit was planned and implemented by my sister. Thankfully, my nephew was there to help, and my aunt (my dad's sister) also went along for the ride. Of course, my mother went, too!

After the visit home, my sister called me and described the experience in detail. To summarize, my dear father was excited to "go home"; however, once he walked into the house he seemed, "disoriented" and actually anxious and uncomfortable. He was like a fish out of water. This was a house that he'd lived in for over forty years, yet it seemed like a strange place to him now. It had been six weeks since he had been there. My sister and I knew that this reaction was related to his stroke and the resultant Left Neglect, as well as his dementia. We figured that what he was seeing did not match his memories. I would guess that things did not appear the same so it must have felt very frightening to him. The result was that he wanted to leave after about fifteen minutes.

He sat at his piano and tried to play and this did not feel the same to him either. His left hand was not doing what it should. Oh, how hard that must have been for my mother to watch and for my father to experience, as well as upsetting for my sister, my aunt and nephew. My sister and I talked about what happened on this visit home and determined together that going home was definitely not the right option. It helped us both to move past any hope of them going back home, which helped us both to face the facts and move forward in the plan to move them. Now, the question was where—an Assisted Living facility in Florida or Michigan?

Florida or Michigan?

My sister immediately followed up on calling and visiting the two or three recommended facilities in Michigan that I had been told about by the social worker where he was living at the time. Based on the really high price per month for the facility he was staying in at the time, we had already hoped that we did not have to keep him there. At the same time, my husband and I searched the Internet and began touring assisted living facilities in Florida during my trip home from Michigan.

At this point of researching and touring potential places in Florida, we didn't fully have a grasp or understand that there were variations of how assisted living was offered and/or provided. My husband and I thought that we had found something very quickly that appeared to be just the perfect place for my parents. We put my parents' names on their waiting list (a very common occurrence, as most places in Florida were found to be full). In the meantime, we looked at a few other places that were converted hotels, which didn't seem very handicap accessible and their layouts were confusing for us when we did our walk-throughs. And, then there were the facilities that seemed really great in just about every way except they offered only two levels of care; independent living and assisted living. We finally stumbled upon a place only fifteen minutes from us that provided all three levels of care: Independent Living, Assisted Living and Skilled Nursing Care. It felt like the best thing possible for our parents.

We knew that my father's medical health was compromised by his brittle diabetes and were concerned about what would happen if he needed to be hospitalized or if my mother needed to be taken out to the hospital. Without a skilled nursing center attached, we knew that it would be difficult for either parent, if one of them needed short or long-term skilled nursing care. Assisted living does not provide such care, and hospitals discharge patients sooner in the this day and age, either sending them home with in-home-health care, or sending them to a "nursing home" type of setting where they can receive things like wound care, IV's, etc.

We discovered this because my experience up in Michigan alerted me to the fragility of my father's health care needs based upon his brittle diabetes. For example, if he needed to go to the hospital again and required follow up skilled nursing care, something that the assisted living could not fulfill, my mother would need to take a taxi alone to visit him. The facility may or may not be equipped to provide a ride to the hospital or skilled nursing facility. This seemed like a very bad set-up for them, so we quickly looked for a place that had all three levels under one "roof," or on the same property. Florida seems more advanced and sophisticated in what they offer; however, there were still many places that did not have this important option. For some people, the two levels of care might work out fine, but for my parents, it would not have been the best type of place to live.

During this time I learned a great deal about what to look for and how to ask the right questions. I found that some places presented well, with beautiful foyers and entrances, but while touring the place, I kept my eyes open for how the residents appeared, and if there were staff members visible and interactive with individuals. I recall one place that had people in the hallways lined up against the walls with nothing stimulating going on at all. Many were sleeping in wheel chairs with nothing to look at and nobody interacting with them. They claimed that they would bring them out, just to get them out of their rooms. This was not near a nursing station and it seemed quite sterile to me and my gut told me that this was not the place for my parents.

I learned to listen to how the place made me feel, not based upon what I saw in a brochure. This approach proved helpful in all of my caregiving experiences that were yet to be experienced. I have found that there are sometimes stereotypes and expectations of the elderly and disabled that can be detrimental to their care. How the nurses' aides understand the needs of the patients can make a huge difference in the care they receive. I look back on my first journey with my parents with a feeling that it was my first "rodeo," but it was the ride I needed to teach me what I needed to know to help others down the road. Each time I had to find the right placement for the family member in need, I learned something new.

An additional issue for my father was access to the administration of insulin injections for his diabetic care. What I found out is that many places, especially in Michigan, there is no staff member, or nurse on site approved to give insulin injections. As a result one should find someone or hire/contract with a nurse from outside of the organization to provide this care. When I share my aunt and uncle's story, I will explain more on this dilemma. Briefly, there does not seem to be a consistent way that this type of need is managed from facility to facility. For my father, we were very fortunate that the place we found for him in Florida provided a nurse on his floor that gave him his shot in his apartment.

Since my first experience in 1999 of moving a person with medical, mental and physical disabilities, the business of assisting our aging population has come a long way. There is so much more accessible information on the internet to help in your quest for the right placement, and it can give you the important knowledge you will need to ask the right questions in your attempt to get the right type of placement for your loved one or friend. There are even television ads for help with finding a home for your elderly parent.

What I learned in the process of researching appropriate placements for my family members:

1. Research ahead of your meeting with any Admissions person. Write down your questions ahead of the meeting.

2. Go on a complete tour of the facility and, if possible, go at different times of day, or at meal times. Many places will invite you for a lunch in the resident dining room. This is very helpful and highly suggested. (The reality is that this isn't always possible if you do not live in the area, and/or cannot travel to where those you are helping live. If possible find someone you know that you trust who lives near your loved one to go tour the place on your behalf. You cannot pick in my opinion based upon a video or brochure.)

3. Go online and read reviews and obtain State inspection statistics and reports.

4. Find out exactly what kind of care is offered in each facility being considered; such as how many levels of care are provided.

5. Take notes while touring.

6. Ask about availability of insulin injections for diabetics. Do they have Extended Congregate Care as an option?

7. Find out how many meals are provided per day. Some are only two, with a snack. We opted for three meals due to my father's diabetes and my parent's inability to organize meals and shopping.

8. Find out what specific kinds of activities are offered/provided. Meet the Activities director if possible.

9. Find out what kind of nursing care is provided. Does the facility have a licensed nurse on duty, or all Certified Nurse's Aides (CNA's)

10. While being interviewed by Admissions, make sure you ask as many questions as you can.

11. Take as much time as you need to make your decision. If feeling rushed by the person taking you on the tour, don't rush through your own opportunity to gather the facts necessary to make an informed decision.

12. If possible, take someone else with you on tour; another family member, or friend. It helps to have two people observing as it is an emotional task for most people, and our ability to remember or view things objectively is not as strong.

13. Before signing anything, make certain to read the fine print and understand exactly the timelines for admission, length of stay, deposit fees and refund qualifications.

When faced with getting things done during a crisis, it can feel insurmountable and unattainable. It is important to take notes when speaking to those who are telling us what steps to take to prepare for moving someone into a care facility, be it a nursing home or an assisted living center. There is so much to cover and most likely our mind will feel cluttered and distracted and filled with a sense that we cannot possibly get everything done in a timely fashion.

For me, there was this internal tug of war over whether or not I should even be moving my parents into a facility. I often felt guilty and went through the mental gymnastics of reviewing all of the reasons why neither I nor my sister or brother could take my parents on our own. This is where we need to learn some ways to relax and take care of ourselves. It can be overwhelming and frightening to say the very least. Change is a challenge for people under the best of circumstances; however, adding all of the ingredients of managing someone else's life changes, while attending to your own life, adds another dimension altogether.

CHAPTER FIVE

THE MOVE TO FLORIDA

The first challenge was that we were placed on a wait list for an assisted-living apartment in Florida. The plan was for my father to stay where he was and continue to receive therapy, with the goal to move him out of skilled nursing care to assisted living care, which would be on a different floor with less medical care and more emphasis on day to day living goals, rehabilitation and socialization. He received three meals per day in the dining room. Here he showed evidence of difficulty finishing his food, due to not seeing the food on his plate. The staff would rotate his plate to ensure that he saw the food he was served. My father wanted to go back home, as so many people do under the same circumstances, but from all recommendations as well as my own observations and knowledge of what "home" was, I knew that he should not go home.

The physician assigned to his care was very honest and straight-forward about my father's prospects for further advancement in his abilities. Her most significant input was the fact that his brain was being most affected by his vascular dementia plus blood sugar problems along with the difficulty to control his diabetes effectively anymore. She did not anticipate that this would get better and warned my sister and me that although he did have the ability to walk, enjoyed his meals still, and perhaps, with time he may be able to play some golf (this was the hope of the physical therapist, and me, too). She bluntly told us that realistically he would not get better in the way that we had hoped for.

Despite this rather pessimistic outlook or prognosis, I took my father to Florida with the goal to help him to enjoy life and get the best care possible for as long as he was able to participate in the things he loved. In Florida, he would continue with therapy to assist him with his transition to his new life and reinforce what they had been working on with him in Michigan. The most important thing I realized was that it was important to take things one day at a time and oftentimes, one step at a time and enjoy the time that he had left with us on earth.

One detail before bringing my parents to Florida that was fun for me was to buy furniture for their new apartment. "Rooms to Go" furniture worked for us; however there is always an option to rent furniture, if you think the time will be short term. I was hopeful that their time would be extended, so I went for purchasing. We actually helped with this expense, as it was clear that my parents needed help until their home sold up in Michigan.

It brought me and my husband joy to see how happy they were when they saw the apartment for the first time and realized it was theirs. I tried to match their taste and they even commented on how much they loved the colors, when they saw the place for the first time. We did ship some familiar paintings from their Michigan home to place in their new "home" that we knew were very sentimental or important to them. We couldn't move their furniture, but pieces of their history were very important for them to have. We made sure there were photographs of family, and other familiar items placed in the apartment.

Moving Day-Fear of the Unknown

First and foremost, thank God I had my nephew to help me move my parents, which involved flying, something my parents rarely did even when they were young and healthy. Their favorite mode of travel was to drive, even from Michigan to Wyoming to visit my sister and family. Their last trip across the country was something we all objected to and tried to convince them to fly not drive; we were unsuccessful. Again, another miraculous uneventful drive that did not end in disaster.

Anyway, prior to this flight to Florida, their most recent experience with flying was with my husband and me to attend my brother-in-law's funeral in February, 1997. With my father and mother's limitations, this newest venture was challenging, but doable. My nephew and I were a good team. We split up so I sat with my father and my nephew sat with my mother on the plane. My father chatted the entire trip. He was excited but also confused. I often had to reorient him throughout the flight as to where we were going and why. The flight was three hours long, so near the end the questions and confusion increased, but we made it!! We were picked up by a service that fit all of us and our luggage into a van. We knew the driver well, and he was the perfect guy to greet my dad for sure. I think my father thought he was being picked up by a limo, making him feel very important.

Fast forward to my parents' introduction to their new home/apartment. The entry into the facility was beautiful and the people at the facility were very welcoming. So far so good, I thought. We took the elevator to their new apartment on the third floor. I knew this was going to take time for them to adjust to. The layout of the building even confused me in the beginning, so I knew it would be really confusing to my parents. Anyway, the driver helped us get the luggage to the apartment, and my husband was also there to greet us and had made the finishing touches on their apartment before we arrived. They were pleasantly receptive to what they saw at first, and didn't say anything negative. However, when my father followed the driver to the door, I saw him say something to him in a whisper. I then followed the driver to the elevator and he told me my father had said to him, "Can you get me out of here? Take me with you!"

So, my father wasn't as happy about his introduction to his new life as I had hoped, but we managed to distract him with a short tour and then I left them to rest and the staff did their admittance exam. Anyone coming into Assisted Living must be physically examined for wounds, bruises, unusual physical attributes; heart and blood pressure and temperature are taken for a baseline. My father was technically the identified patient at this point.

I liken the dropping off of my parents to their new home with dropping off a child at school for the first time. I knew it would be a huge adjustment and that they would have many feelings related to this life change. I tried to balance my early involvement and visits to provide support, but not hover or take over things for them. They needed to learn the ropes, and how to get help from the staff. I was anxious myself and felt so bad about everything that had yet to happen. I had to continue to travel to Michigan to help my nephew get ready for the sale of the house.

Prior to moving my parents, I was able to get hold of an old friend who was a realtor to sign the contracts to put the house on the market. I did have my parents participate in this process and the realtor/friend was the perfect guy for the job. His family was well-known and trusted in my parent's town and my father had known of his father. This helped considerably with my father's ability to trust him. With his tendency toward denial (in fact my sister and I affectionately called him the "King of De-Nile"), the thought of selling his home was not easy for him at all. The realtor's gift of gab and "guys'/guy" personality helped smooth the waters and we actually got his blessing to sell. Phew! Yes, I had the authority with my Powers to sell the property, but I wanted my parents to have a part in the process as a way to give them their dignity. To rip away all of their independence would have been wrong!! If he had opposed the decision, I could have legally overridden him with my Powers of Attorney that were already in effect.

Fortunately, they adjusted to their new "home." They loved the balcony that they had. My father enjoyed the Florida sunshine and sitting and watching people come and go through the front entrance of the facility. Life suddenly became much simpler for my parents and this was a good thing.

Legal Issues

Once in, Florida, there were many adjustments and details to be attended to by me as my parents' Power of Attorney and Patient Advocate. Legal concerns that were handled in MI, along with financial issues had to be taken care of again in Florida. I closed all bank accounts in Michigan, and then reopened accounts in Florida. The facility that my parents moved into actually had a satellite bank within the building, which was very convenient, and they also had a financial advisor. Fortunately, my husband sat in and reviewed what was being recommended, and with his financial planning background, he recommended that we not go with the advice given, which was high risk and not good for someone of their age.

The lesson here is make sure you don't jump to things with any big financial changes based upon one recommendation. Conservative conservation of funds for my parents was the best option. At this point, my parents' house had just been put on the market and had not yet sold. I found it a disconcerting how quickly a financial advisor moved in with an aggressive investment plan for my parents. This is how seniors are oftentimes duped into making some very bad financial decisions. In my parents' case, we knew that they were going to need access to their money for their care, and to tie it up was not a sound option.

Luckily, we were able to use our Michigan attorney for my father in Florida. He practiced in south Florida and Michigan, and to top it off, his father was still the figurehead senior partner of the Law firm, whom my father happened to know very well from his fifty years practicing in Michigan. My father was excited to go to his office, because he would see a familiar person professionally from our hometown. This helped to get over the hurdle of once again looking at end of life planning, which my father had avoided like the plague most of his life. He wanted to wear a suit and tie to go to the meeting and he comported himself with dignity and professionalism and was able to fake his way through things, appearing quite well.

The experience exhausted him, but it was such a wonderful way to empower my father again, who had lost so much of his liberty and abilities over a short period of time. This meeting gave me a sense of pride for my dad, and I felt so grateful for this serendipity to have come in the beginning of my parents' time in Florida. We needed to get this all done quickly, and I had already made the appointment prior to the move of my parents, so everything was drawn up before I took my parents in to sign the paperwork.

We updated the wills and powers of attorney to be legal in Florida and my parents were able to sign the paperwork and feel like participating adults. After feeling so impotent with respect to the move, their physical health and consequent changes and the scariness of not remembering things or knowing where they were, this visit to the lawyer's office was actually uplifting to both of my parents. In other words, we put a positive spin on things and included them in decision making where and whenever we could. Again, this is important to try to achieve, whenever you can as a caregiver.

Adjusting to a New Life

My parents' adjustment to their new life was not easy, but all-in-all they adapted quite well all things considered. They loved having their eleven year old cat with them. She was very special to my parents and something they could take care of. People would come to visit my parents simply to see "Winnie" the cat. This gave my parents great enjoyment. When I looked for the right assisted living place for my parents, one of my primary pre-requisites was the place must be pet friendly. Fortunately, I found one that was, because many are not.

It was a big relief for me to watch my parents become comfortable in their apartment and settle into a routine. My parents were people who liked routine, so this fit their personalities. And, with their memory issues, this was certainly the best formula for success. All of their needs were being met, so for me, this was very comforting. I knew their risks had reduced considerably from when they were living alone in their own home. The benefits of the move far outweighed the negatives. Despite their loss of their life in Michigan, they were now in a safer environment, their needs were being taken care of and their stress level reduced considerably compared to the life they were living before the crisis. I enjoyed having them both nearby so we could spend quality time together.

All Is Well At First

My father's day-to-day medical needs were met by the facility doctor who managed their general health with visits to their apartment on a scheduled basis. I believe it was once a month that he would stop in and take their blood pressures and listen to their heart and talk to them for a bit. The point of this is that they were monitored frequently, which was good. Periodically, my father had erratic blood sugars, which resulted in episodes requiring medical intervention. It was a relief to know that my parents were no longer on their own anymore. Having them being taken care of was reassuring to all of us.

The downside of this care is that it is not always reliable, and different staff members can make all the difference in the world. Some were kind hearted and really caring toward my parents and some would barely speak to them. Fortunately, the nursing supervisor was top notch and she loved my parents. My parents remembered her name always, even if they couldn't remember if they had eaten lunch yet. She was special, which as I found throughout my years of caregiving, makes all the difference in the world.

Living nearby, I was able to participate in taking my parents to doctor's appointments when necessary. One essential treatment that my father needed was for his "diabetic retinopathy," to hopefully improve or retain his eyesight. Diabetic retinopathy is a disease of the eye that can blur vision and destroy the retina. It is commonly associated with diabetes. We would drive almost an hour each way to get my father's treatments, which I would schedule for him. Each time we went my mother would marvel that I could find my way around so well. Getting the treatments would hopefully help my father continue to golf. His driving days were already over.

Even with poor eyesight we had some fun and successful golf outings together. My mother had been a golfer, too, so we would all go together. There was a golf center with five courses near the facility where they lived.

I would take them over for lunch followed by playing as many holes as they could handle. Doing a full nine wasn't easy, but we tried in the beginning. After some time, we found a par 3 that was near my house. It was shorter and easier and both parents could enjoy this experience. My father couldn't see very well, but he had incredible muscle memory from his years of golfing; his favorite pastime and obsession. I actually had to tee up his ball for him, point him in the right direction and then he would swing and make contact with the ball just about every time. It still brings tears to my eyes as I remember how happy that made him feel. I would describe his ball flight and clap when he hit it well.

One day he said to me while we were golfing, "Why are you so nice to me?"

I kiddingly said, "I have no idea, Dad!"

We both laughed, but then I said that I loved him and wanted to give back some of what he gave me. The thing about this was that we both knew he was not an easy-going Dad, and his emphasis was with my brother growing up, not me. We did not talk about this, but I did tell him that I always knew he loved me and that's what mattered most. He was a tough father, like so many from my era, and I felt that any feelings I had at that point were trumped by my desire to help make the end of his life meaningful and enjoyable as best as possible. I saw him do it for his parents and for my mom's mother, and my mother was always good to her in-laws (my grandparents) as well. I believe such positive role modeling stuck with me. I cherish having the opportunity to spend this kind of time with my parents in their "sunset years."

I made time for my parents to help them settle into their new lives. I found it hard to leave them, much like leaving a kid at school for the first time, hoping that they would adjust. The staff was great, and my father seemed to enjoy the social aspect of the atmosphere. He was always a gregarious person and this remained a strength for him; a true blessing. The nurses and aides and food staff loved both of my parents, which helped everything go more smoothly. They seemed to understand my father's volatility when it showed up and they handled him well, especially in the beginning.

During my parents' first summer in Florida, I was lucky in that that I was able to travel to Michigan, as was our custom, because my parents had settled in nicely since moving into their Assisted Living apartment in February of 2000. My aunt and uncle (my mother's brother) and my sister all visited my parents during my absence. I also called my parents every single day that I was away. During their first spring in Florida, my dad's previous law partner and his wife came to stay about only thirty minutes from where my parents were, which was wonderful, because they would visit my parents while they were down for lunch and catching up. They had not seen this couple for years, as they had moved to the east coast, so when we figured out that they could get together with such great friends, it was just perfect for everyone involved. I enjoyed orchestrating and organizing these visits for everyone and found that my willingness to reach out and communicate and plan made all the difference and my family was nice enough to let me know how much they appreciated my help. I am not telling this to brag, but to point out the importance of someone helping those they are caring for to stay connected with people in their lives, which they no longer can organize for themselves.

And, good things did happen in their new residence. Whenever I visited them at the apartment, somebody very often came up to me to tell me that they loved my parents. Staff actually commented that my parents were polite and treated staff with respect. Apparently, this wasn't always the case with residents. I remember feeling proud to be their daughter. It was very sad for me to see my dad decline day by day in his abilities. He had some good days and some bad days. I admired his tenacity and desire to try to get better, and I think for him, in some way it was a blessing that he didn't fully comprehend his new limitations. Yes, with his inability to remember or grasp that he had left neglect, it was a health and safety risk always, but he was able to adapt enough to function fairly well.

One thing that was certain was that they were both in the right place by being in assisted living and in Florida near my husband and me. We were able to enjoy holidays with them along with my husband's mother and his sister and son, who also lived in the area. I remember their first Easter in Florida, where we all went to brunch. My father was in his element. He dressed in a suit and seemed so happy. This was about two months into his time in Florida. He needed assistance, and at this point was receptive to help from me. We brought them to our home for other holidays, and both parents really enjoyed this as well.

I could see my dad making progress early on and so I held on to much hope for more improvement along the way. We got them a mailbox, and he and my mother were able to get their mail each day, which was very important to their sense of independence. My mother and he oftentimes did this together, which increased their chances of finding the box and handling the key to open it. We got them clips for the door key and PO Box key to hang on their belt loops. This works very well. And, in fact, they had already started this habit on their own before my father's stroke, as a way for them to compensate for their failing memories.

By the way, from my observation over the years, most elderly living in facilities like this love to get their mail; sometimes they go multiple times in a day, forgetting they have already done so earlier. It can be a nice way for socialization to occur, too. My parents loved talking to the people at the front desk on their trips down to the lobby.

Another great opportunity for my father for positive social interaction and enjoyment, was for him to go down to the lobby where there was a grand piano. From the time I saw this piano on my first tour of the place, I thought and hoped that this might be a great opportunity for him. He loved playing the organ and piano before his stroke and I wasn't sure how he would do afterward. Well, what happened when he saw the piano was so heartwarming and amazing to me at the same time. He walked up to it and hit a couple of keys and I encouraged him to sit down and play. His memory of one of his favorite songs was not lost and he began to play quite well, considering his left hand was not fully engaged. Nonetheless, the song was recognizable and people stopped to listen and watch. The business offices for the facility were next to this lobby. Office staff came out and clapped for my father and also complimented him and he beamed with happiness. He was always a ham, so this could not have been a better experience for him early on in his stay at his new "home." All in all, my father adjusted to his new life and actually adapted quite well. Both of my parents thrived with the extra care and attention and they enjoyed the social aspect of the facility in the beginning.

The Michigan doctor from the Skilled Nursing facility in Michigan warned us that his behavior may get worse as his impulse control, memory, judgment and tolerance for change would also deteriorate. She explained to my sister and me that one of the common conditions cited as a cause of vascular dementia is diabetes. Her words cut like a knife. I did not want to hear what she was saying, but I never forgot what she said, and nor did my sister. In retrospect, this doctor's honesty helped us to accept what was happening, when my father's overall day-to-day functioning ultimately changed for the worse. My hopes for my father making a good recovery under the right care were dashed. However, I continued to hope for better things for both my parents with their new life and set out to provide the best opportunity for them to have as good a life as they could under the circumstances.

One concern early on in their time in the new assisted living apartment was that my father had a tendency to wander once he was feeling better physically. He always seemed to have a knack for luck his entire life, which definitely came in handy here.

There were two times that I remember where his disorientation could have gotten him into terrible trouble. One time, he decided to walk to the strip mall near their facility to buy a thermometer for their small balcony so that he could know the temperature outside. He always loved thermometers. He managed to find his way there, but then could not find his way back. A stranger picked him up and somehow figured out where he lived and brought him back to the lobby. This happened one other time as well. The second time he "escaped," he returned with only one shoe. This time, a taxi brought him back to the facility. I imagine that people in the area were familiar with this sort of thing happening, because at this point, he was not in a lock down area, so he could sign out or just walk out. The front desk people learned this about my dad and the staff became more aware of his comings and goings.

In the beginning, my father's insulin and sugar levels were managed quite well, thanks to the consistent administration of his injections, because of the nursing service on their floor. He would sit at the nurses' desk every day, starting about one hour before he needed the shot, just to make sure they didn't forget him. He still knew he needed the shot and being controlling, he was proactive in getting it, which was a good thing. It gave him a sense of participation and engagement in his self-care, which was very important to his self-esteem. Wherever independence can be maintained is essential to try to foster and encourage. It can be a fine line to achieve due to safety issues, but for my parents, much easier in a self-contained facility, which actually encourage independence as much as possible for the residents. If you have a loved one in a facility that doesn't encourage this, you should intervene in some way to see what can be done to improve this aspect of their care.

At night, my father's need for supervision increased. He would get disoriented and end up in other people's apartments, or wandering the halls, without his clothing. Medical intervention helped to stop this problem, as did the fact that he became more oriented over time to his surroundings. The term, "sundowning," is often used to describe the phenomena with the elderly where their confusion and tendency to wake up during the evening, or not be able to sleep at all. Besides the confusion and restlessness, it includes wandering off and being combative. As staff got to know my father, they were able to help with such symptoms with medications, changes in activities and other techniques. If you are a caregiver at home, there are many good suggestions on the internet to help with this issue. And, most importantly, of course, consult medical personnel who can design a management plan to help your loved one and you.

CHAPTER SIX

ONE YEAR LATER:
THE DOWNWARD SPIRAL IS RAPID

When my parents first arrived in the Florida facility, even though he was on an Assisted Living floor, equipped with a small private dining area, they were given the opportunity to go downstairs to the large dining area where most of the people were from the Independent Living floors. It was like eating in a restaurant, which they both loved. My husband and I also took them out to lunches and dinners quite frequently. And, in the beginning he did well with this, but over a period of time things changed for the worse. It was decided at some point that my father and mother could not manage being in the large dining room. My parents both were having difficulty handling the confusion that came with waiting for the doors to open, and they would go down too soon and my father would become agitated and impatient. It was good to give them a chance to try it in the beginning, but when it was time to downsize to the small on floor dining room, we had an option already available for them. This setting was just down the hall from them and provided more oversight and assistance where needed. My father settled into this change very well.

Things were starting to become more and more difficult for my father with respect to his daily living skills, and his mental confusion was getting worse. I recall my feeling disappointed and once again trying to find what external forces and causes might be at play or to blame.

As the secondary caregiver, I felt like a failure when my father's behavior and capabilities were going downhill, even though my rational brain reminded me that this was to be expected. Nonetheless, I kept fighting for him to get better! This was the desire to "help people" coming out; not a bad thing, but when we are very close to someone, it is more likely that we won't see things as they are at times. In other words, we can lose our objectivity.

This is where it was helpful for me to talk to my family members, who were not there day in and day out. I would get their input when I felt that I was not happy with what was going on. I also made a point to ask questions of the professionals caring for my father. Yes, sometimes it is intimidating to ask questions, and we may not like the answers we get, or the attitude of the person we are asking questions, but it is important to forge ahead and ask away. We have a right to ask and, as an advocate for the person we are responsible for, it is one of the most important aspects of your role.

A Danger to Himself and Others

My father did fairly well when he first moved to Florida and he reaped the benefits of having family nearby and very attentive care with three meals served a day, along with stimulating activities; however, he started to show signs of significant mental and physical decline after about one year. And, once this happened, the changes were rapid and not easily managed. On top of this, he became a danger to himself and others; specifically, my mother. One of the first times I received a call regarding my father's behavior was after a trip to a restaurant on the facility bus, with a group of other residents. He became extremely belligerent and out of control in the public restaurant, creating quite a scene. The degree of his volatility had increased lately, but the staff still thought a trip out might be good for him and my mother. Yes, we had been taking them to dinners, but this was different. The unpredictability of the setting, the lack of individual attention and his increasing disorientation and confusion were a bad combination. Medications were prescribed and his behavior was followed after this episode.

The next time that I was called in the middle of the night regarding my father's behavior, I became extremely concerned, but also a bit doubtful of the reports given by the staff. Frankly, it was very hard to accept what they were telling me about his unmanageable wandering and outbursts. I hoped that as long as I was available to take the staff calls, and confer with the doctors, that we would be able to keep him with my mother in their apartment, on the assisted living floor. Unfortunately, this was no longer possible.

One night my father became violent with my mother, and the staff were frightened that she could get hurt, so they took my father out of their apartment immediately and placed him downstairs into the nursing home section of the facility. I remember being thankful that we had found a facility with all three levels of care so that he was not taken out of the building to another place where it would have been difficult for my mother to be able to visit him. What this move did lead to, however, was a rapid decline in functioning. Yes, the changes were already happening, but to me the fact that he was swept away from my mother in the middle of the night added to his confusion and I was not happy about how the whole thing unfolded. However, they were probably right. I just wished they had called me sooner so that I could have spoken to him over the phone.

Dad Not Safe

At this point, the wheels were now in motion for the downward spiral of my dad's ability to live with my mother anymore. It was very sad for me to see this happening. In all honesty it wasn't a total surprise, but our minds do not want to accept things like this and so we rationalize behaviors and deny what we are seeing before us. Yes, intellectually I knew that we had bought him some quality time, where he didn't have to live with so much stress anymore, but I still felt so responsible somehow for his not doing better. This was not rational, and I understood it afterward, but in the middle of this experience I was not always able to accept the changes that were happening. The end of my father's life was not easy for him or those around him.

My Father Looked and Acted "Crazy"

The next morning I drove up to the facility to see my mother first, and then to visit my father in the nursing home downstairs. To go into the nursing home section, you had to go through two large doors. I was not sure what I would find once inside and I was feeling very nervous. Upon entering, I saw the circular nursing station, with a few nurses standing there. As I approached them, I noticed my father in an odd looking chair on wheels, within the circle of the nursing station itself. He was below the desk shelving so I couldn't see him at first, but I heard him shout my name, "Lin," very loudly, he looked panicky and trapped. He was dangerously trying to climb out of what looked like a high chair of sorts with wheels. It was restraining my father, so that he couldn't walk himself, as he was a risk for a fall and for escape. He was extremely disruptive. I was shocked and frightened by what I saw and so angry that he was being treated like this. I wanted to talk to the person in charge right away. I was literally shaking physically and asked to speak to the supervisor. My father was very agitated!

He was calling out my mother's name and asked me where she was. I told him that I would bring her down very shortly after I spoke to his doctor. He continued shouting out my mothers' name over and over.

I needed to know more about the episode that got him into this situation before bringing my mother downstairs to see him. What I found out is that he had physically pushed my mother and was "out of control." They had medicated him, but as I could see, he was still very excitable and scared. In my estimation he seemed terrified and unable to understand what was happening to him.

The scene actually reminded me of my days working in a Day Treatment Center for Emotionally Impaired children, who were sometimes explosive and had to be restrained and contained in the school office. As the social worker I was called upon to help calm the student and redirect their anger in a more productive and less disruptive way. The skills I had learned actually came in handy with my father. I was able to speak to him and he did calm down, but only when I was by his side. When I left, he panicked and began shouting again. I felt so helpless and very sad seeing my father like this.

Here I was observing my father at the age of eighty, an adult with be-havior seen in a two- year-old. This was so distressing. I wanted to cry, but instead I actually felt angry. For me personally this was a typical reaction for me. Rather than cry, I wanted to fight to make things right. Fortunately, I knew how important it was for me to keep my anger in check, so that I could help my father by getting to a place where I could be assertive in my requests for information, without yelling at anyone, or making a scene. I needed to be his advocate, not his irrational daughter demanding answers. I managed to keep my cool and knew that jumping to conclusions would not be helpful, and that I must ask valid and appropriate questions of those in charge.

My emotions were running high, which made it more difficult to main-tain my own self-control. For example, the nurses looked completely fed up with having to "babysit" my father, and I felt their steely stares. Whether or not they actually looked at me this way is debatable, but that's how it felt. I felt embarrassed, even though I knew his dementia, the stroke he had the year before, along with his medical condition were at the root of this behavior. Nonetheless, it's like when a kid acts out in a store and the parent feels all eyes staring at them as their child has a temper tantrum. Only this time, it was me the adult child, feeling embarrassed by their parent; a very uncomfortable role reversal for sure.

I asked a nurse sitting at the nurses' station if I could please speak to the Supervisor. She barely looked up at me and said she'd see if she was available. The supervisor's office was kitty corner from the nurses' station. She glanced up and noted her door was closed, so it might be a bit before I could speak to her. Meanwhile, my father was shouting out my mother's name over and over, and asking where she was. He saw me and shouted, "Get me out of here," over and over. I was feeling so helpless and I felt my anger getting stronger by the minute. In a situation like this, it is not unusual to feel this way. What was happening to my father was the most important thing to me in that moment. For the nurse, this kind of thing happens routinely with dementia patients. For me it was personal, for her, it was part of her job. I "got that" but when we're in the moment, it is very hard to keep things in perspective.

I felt like yelling and screaming. Instead, I dug deep and made a conscious decision to remain assertive and polite in asking if there was anyone else that I could speak to in private about my father's condition. My assertiveness did lead to the result I wanted. As soon as the supervisor was free, she came out and brought me into her office to talk. She was receptive to my questions and answered them as best she could. At this point, their goal was to keep my father safe, while under their care, but they could not keep him with his behaviors. They had ordered a psychiatric consultation. I can't recall how long it took, but before long, my father was taken by ambulance to the local hospital that had a psychiatric unit. I recall it being on the seventh floor.

I followed him to the hospital and helped the staff there collect important background information, much like the social histories I used to do for the children that I helped or evaluated. If my memory serves me, the first person I met with was a social worker. My father required sedation and did not even look like the father I knew, and he was acting very strangely.

My premise was that when they had to take my father away from my mother in the middle of the night and move him down to the nursing home section of their facility, he completely fell apart, or "decompensated." He could not cope without my mother, and at this point, he still had not seen her. My goal was to share what I thought might help my father and to ask how we could make this happen.

The Need for Psychiatric Hospitalization

Things happened quickly once it was decided that my father should not stay in the Skilled Nursing section of his facility, because he had behaved aggressively toward my mother in their assisted living apartment and had been unmanageable and extremely agitated. He was placed in the psychiatric ward of a nearby hospital, which lucky for me was only a half-mile from my home. The staff who called the ambulance, felt and stated that my father was at risk of hurting himself and/or others. Because of this, and because my father was unable to make the decisions for himself at this time, I was asked to become his Temporary Legal Guardian. The recommendation was for my father to remain on the seventh floor for observation for a seventy-two hour period.

The term Baker Act is a Florida Mental Health Act. In my father's case the Baker Act was intended to admit him for an involuntary observation/examination period with treatment. The goal was to return him to his "community," or home as soon as possible. I was provided a private area to watch a video regarding Guardianship re: what my role would be. After I watched I signed forms agreeing to be his guardian. At this point, my guardianship was considered to be temporary. I felt really conflicted. He needed to be placed in an environment for observation and to ensure his safety as well as those around him; however, I hated seeing him in a psychiatric hospital setting. It was all so distressing!

I was feeling overwhelmed by this charge and remember questioning so many things at the time. I decided to reach out to my sister to run everything by her before signing or agreeing to anything. I didn't usually feel so ambivalent or uncertain, but everything seemed to be thrown at me so quickly. I did not want to do anything to harm my father, and I understood that he needed help, but I needed someone else to support my decisions and reassure that I was doing the right thing. Trusting our own judgment can be clouded by the stress of watching someone we love, and who has always been the person in charge, fall apart psychologically. My sister agreed to come to be with my mother, while I handled all of the daily crises that seemed to be rolling in fast and furiously. Frequent phone calls and frequent meetings with doctors seemed to run my days for a while. My sister coming in was welcomed and needed.

Within the first seventy-two hours, my father's behavior and physical health deteriorated. I was afraid we would lose him in the hospital and that he would never make it back "home." My professional background told me that this was best for him, but I kept finding myself trying to find what external trigger caused this shift in behavior. I knew intellectually that his brain was effected by his stroke and his brittle diabetes, but because of my own denial that things were going downhill, I wanted to blame the way the facility handled his removal from my mom in the middle of the night. The good thing was that he could be evaluated medically and psychiatrically and I knew this, but at first I was feeling that the system had failed all of us. The bottom line was that my father's dementia and physical problems were getting worse. I needed to find it in my heart to trust the decision made, but this did not mean that I did not need to stay involved and be a part of the process. I also needed to be there for my mother, who certainly needed emotional support during this tumultuous and confusing time for her and my father.

His medical problems as well as his behavioral issues were reportedly not easy for the staff to regulate or manage. Medications were prescribed along with close monitoring. I arranged to take my mother to go visit him as soon as I was given the green light by the "powers that be." I wanted to make sure that the visit would not be too stressful for my mother, and I wanted to make sure that the hospital staff felt it would be a positive thing for my father. I was given the go-ahead and I drove my mother to go for our first visit. It was a terrible feeling to be going to see my father in a psychiatric ward. I dreaded going and tried to remain upbeat for my mother, while we drove to the hospital together in the car. I know we were both nervous. For my mother, it was a lot to take in and process. It was all difficult. She had been the target of my father's irrational anger and physical aggression—the reason behind his being removed from their apartment in the first place. Then they were unable to go back "home" after he could not be controlled in the nursing home section of their facility. So she had every right to be confused.

"You Did This to Me"

One of my worst memories of my father's time in the psychiatric facility was the first time I talked to him over the phone when he was an inpatient. When I called him to tell him I was there with mom, the first words out of his mouth were, "Get me out of here…you did this to me, you put me here, now get me out of here." That's all I remember he would say to me. I tried to explain to him that the doctors made the decision but that I thought it was a good plan, because he was in need of help.

Our first visit together with my father was in his room. When we reached the door, we saw my father wandering around his room standing up wearing just a diaper. I remember having a physical reaction to what I was seeing. I had a lump in my throat and I felt embarrassed for him; although he seemed oblivious to his situation, most likely due to the medication he was receiving to keep him sedated. The main aspect of this visit that I want to share is that it was something that I never imagined seeing and I felt so unprepared. You might think that my professional background would prepare me for this situation, but honestly, it did not prepare me for my own feelings and reactions. One part of me wanted to get my father dressed and take him out of the place. The more rational side knew that I needed to speak to his psychiatrist and/or the social worker to get a better understanding of my father's condition and prognosis and his treatment plan and this is what I set out to do. What I found out was that the plan was to stabilize his behaviors with regulating his blood sugars and medications to get him to the point where he could return to the Skilled Nursing Facility. This all sounded like a good and reasonable plan to me. In the meantime, I continued to worry about what I could see was a rapid change in my father's overall health and functioning. What happened next was very telling and really opened my eyes to what was not easy for me to face.

Dysphagia

Early on in my father's stay in the psychiatric unit he had an episode where he choked while in the dining room. He reportedly fell to the floor off of his chair, choking to the point that he stopped breathing. A "Code Blue" alert occurred, meaning that it was severe enough that his heart had stopped beating along with pulmonary distress. My father received CPR, and was successfully resuscitated and sent down to the medical floor emergency room. As the contact person in case of an emergency and as his Patient Advocate I was called and asked to come to the hospital. I went straight from home to the hospital. I felt that until I knew more, I would not worry my mother yet; however, I did call the nurse on my mother's floor back at the facility to let her know what had happened and that I would fill them in once I knew more.

What I found out later was that this first choking episode would be the beginning of my father's diagnosed difficulty with swallowing food, medically termed "dysphagia." The term I began to hear was that my father was aspirating, which means that food and even just saliva does not get swallowed properly and ends up infiltrating the lungs. In my father's case, his swallowing difficulty was one of the effects of his stroke, dementia and aging. The muscles were not able to activate the swallowing mechanism properly and the message to the brain was not functioning as it should. The end result was choking or collection of material in the lungs, which often causes pneumonia. Eating can actually be a painful process as a result. (There is a plethora of information regarding stroke and dementia and Dysphagia on the Internet. I would suggest that you consider researching this on your own if someone you know is experiencing swallowing difficulty.)

By the time I was called by the hospital staff they told me my father had been released from the ER and had been evaluated in the Cardiac Care Unit. When I arrived, he had already been transferred to the fourth floor but I couldn't find him. When I couldn't find him it added to my feelings of helplessness and worry. When they told me where he had been moved, the staff person called the floor by a name I had never heard before. I asked for them to repeat the word, which they did and I still couldn't get what they were saying. I figured the most important information was the floor number, so started to the elevators to find my father on the fourth floor.

Before I sat down to write this part of my father's story, I called the hospital where my father was a patient back fourteen years ago and asked for the fourth floor nurses' station. I briefly explained that I wanted to know the name of the unit. She initially answered that it was called, "Progressive Care." I explained that my father was a patient there in 2001, and I was trying to remember the other name that they used when he was placed there for care after a code blue. She had a heavy accent so it took me a minute to understand the word she said, which was "telemetry." Researching further I found out that recovering cardiac patients requiring monitoring of vital signs, but who no longer require being in the Cardiac Care Unit, are placed in a unit that may be called Progressive or Intermediate Care as a step before a general inpatient setting. In my father's case, he was either in the emergency room or in ICU for a short time and then transferred to the Telemetry floor or the "Telemetry Care Unit." My point in bringing this up, is that the fact that after all these years I still was wondering what in the world the name of the floor was where they put my father after his near death experience. Back in 2001, I remember feeling bugged by not understanding what the nurse was saying, and having no idea what the name meant, yet I gave up on asking and figured it didn't matter, as long as I could find my father.

This story is to encourage you to ask questions, no matter how dumb you might think the questions might be. It's okay not to know, and it is very much okay to ask the professionals or staff members what they mean by something that they have told you about your family member, or the definition of something if you've never heard it before. This is something we've been taught at a young age in school i.e. ask questions, but for some reason, as a caregiver, I found myself sometimes uneasy or unsure of myself and I didn't always ask questions when I should have. Maybe this is or was true for you, too? Possible reasons we don't ask may be that we do not want to appear stupid. Or, we are so overwhelmed by our emotions, that we are not thinking as clearly as we typically might in our day-to-day lives.

Back to what happened next. After I hung up the phone, I immediately drove to the hospital to go visit my father and to get more information about his condition and to find out what the next step would be for him. I was very shocked by the call and very scared about what I might find when I got to the hospital. I assumed that my father would be in Intensive Care, but that was not the case. I stopped by the nurses' station upon arrival to the fourth floor to ask what room he was in. They took me to a large open area where my father was sitting in a recliner type chair right in the middle of the room. He was not in his own room in a bed. He had machines around him with wires attached to him, which were monitoring his vital signs twenty four seven, with monitors placed everywhere in case anything changed in heart rate, etc. Once he was medically stabilized he was returned to the psychiatric ward until medications stabilized his behavior. He was then transferred back to the nursing home, not to the assisted living apartment with my mother, but into the nursing home section.

It's Who You Know

As luck would have it, the psychiatrist at the hospital to whom my father was assigned happened to be a friend of a friend's brother. I was attending a get-together at my friend's house and was introduced to a woman, whose last name was the same as the psychiatrist treating my father. She was also a doctor—not a psychiatrist, but a plastic surgeon. Upon introductions, when I heard her last name, I asked if she knew the doctor. "Sure," she said, "he's my little brother." Today, she and I remain very good friends. That evening she and I talked about our families and got to know one another. She was my age and we had a lot in common. One thing that stands out is how she patiently listened to my tale about my parents and my moving them down to Florida.

Long story short, I was having trouble with the social worker at the nursing home assigned to my father's care, who worked with her brother, my father's psychiatrist. I shared my frustration and she encouraged me to call him and let him know what was happening. I felt the medication he was on to control his behavior was too strong and that my father was not doing well back at the nursing home. His swallowing issues had worsened and he was not getting any better. I wondered if his difficulty swallowing was exacerbated by his medications. My friend's encouragement and suggestions sounded like a good idea so I did call the next day to set up an appointment with the psychiatrist. He told me he, "knew my father's type," the golfer, the lawyer, and that he could talk to him and meet him at his home facility and then he'd follow up with me.

This assessment was done because of my willingness to speak up and reach out to someone whom I thought might be able to better help my father. My being there as an advocate, or in other words an interested family member, definitely made a difference in my father's treatment. This was the beginning of my knowing how important it is to stay involved, ask questions and not be afraid to say something if we do not like what we see or how a family member is doing, or being treated, no matter how intimidating it may feel.

My follow up appointment with the psychiatrist was in his office. It was very productive, and I am glad that I had the opportunity to voice my concerns. Meeting his sister and becoming her friend, still fifteen years later, always amazes me with its timing in my life. Serendipity like this experience seemed to happen in each one of my caregiving situations. I find that sharing with people a bit of what you may have happening to you in your life can open doors and link you to people who can potentially help you.

They may know of resources that we may not. Opening our hearts, ears, and minds can be very helpful in the long run. There is some risk in doing this, but what I find is that if it isn't the right timing or the right person to be of help, we will know pretty quickly and can change the subject to something less personal.

The End of Life Is Near

It was clear that my father's life was coming to an end. It was time to begin to prepare for that day. A side story of importance here is that it was now June, and my husband and I were preparing to head to our cottage in Michigan. In addition to getting our place opened, we needed to check on my parents' place up there as well. It was already about two weeks or more past when we normally went to Michigan, so I was feeling anxious to go. My dilemma was that I didn't want to leave before I was sure my father's issues were settled; however, my husband wanted to go and have me with him to settle in and then fly back within a week or if necessary sooner to be with my parents. Once again, I called upon my sister to spell me during this process. She was completing her semester in her Divinity program and thought she could come and take over for a bit.

Before agreeing to leave, I questioned the doctors about my father's prognosis. To me, he seemed especially fragile and frankly near death. He was still having difficulty with swallowing and he would not open his eyes to look at me during my visits with him. I do remember that he would open his eyes for a second or two and promptly shut them. The doctors assured me that he was not near death and that it was fine for me to leave for a week or so and then come back if I felt I needed or wanted to. Once again I relied on my sister for help. Over the years that I was the "front" person as the family caregiver, I found that despite differences in opinions at times, she and I improved in our communications. We learned each time and although the conflict and tension continued, we grew in our ability to respect one another's opinions and perceptions.

I was terribly worried when I got in the car with my husband and two cats to begin our three-day trek north to Michigan. I called my sister every day and talked to her and my mother. Before I left I connected with all of the staff and professionals to alert them that I was leaving and to get the best handle that I could on my father's status and condition. I felt comfortable with the staff in the nursing home. My mother had good assistance in place and they assured me that they would help her visit my father in the nursing home downstairs. My sister was on her way and would take over where I left off. In the meantime, thanks to cell phones, I could be reached wherever I was.

Before leaving I organized the following:

- Discharge from the hospital,

- Review of my father's Advanced Directives to make sure that his wishes were clear,

- Making sure the "Do Not Resuscitate" order was still in place, valid and appropriate,

- Participating in a care planning meeting with the full staff of those who would be working with my father, and

- Going over everything with my sister. She was the second in line assigned as my parents' Health Care Surrogate, sometimes called a Patient Advocate, depending upon the state.

There are two primary kinds of advance directives: A **living will** spells out your preferences about certain kinds of life-sustaining treatments. For example, you can indicate whether you do or do not want interventions such as cardiac resuscitation, tube feeding, and mechanical respiration; a **power of attorney** directive names someone that you trust to act as your agent if you are unable to speak for yourself. If you want to choose one person to speak for you on health care matters, and someone else to make financial decisions, you can do separate financial and health care powers of attorney. A power of attorney may be more flexible, since it's impossible to predict all the medical decisions that might come up in the future and spell out your exact preferences for all of these situations.

Many states actually combine the living will and power of attorney into one "advance directive" form. Only assign power to someone trusted to make the medical decisions needed to carry out your wishes. For example, your husband or daughter might find it painful to comply with your preference not to have a breathing tube inserted. My suggestion is that you find out what is needed to legally obtain the right to help with medical and mental health decisions when a loved one is unable to do so for themselves. There is plenty of information on the Internet and there are many eldercare attorneys who are well informed.

CHAPTER SEVEN

THE END OF HIS LIFE

The end of my father's life was not easy for all family members. My brother was on the opposite coast in California; not being with my father was difficult as was also true of my father's sister. As a result, I made certain to keep them both up-to-date and in the loop on what was happening with my father's quick decline, as well as include them in the process of trying to make the right end-of-life decisions. They needed to trust the judgment of my sister and me and we needed this support as well. It is always hard to make decisions surrounding life and death. To shut family members out is not helpful in the long run, even if it may seem easier not to contact everyone and just go ahead and follow the Advanced Directives and do what you know or think is best.

In this case, the one thing that seemed to help, was that my brother had come for a short visit. During his visit, I witnessed one of my father's worst moments of confusion and disorientation, while riding down the elevator with my brother and father.

He turned to my brother and said, "Where are you from?"

My brother answered, "California." My brother shrugged and looked at me with a questioning look.

My dad then said, "Really, that's a coincidence, that's where my son lives." We both went with it and didn't make a big deal. We continued the conversation a bit further, but did not point out to him that this is your son. It didn't seem like the right thing to do at that point.

When the elevator doors opened and we got off, my father seemed to reorient when I said to him, "Isn't it great to have John here with us, dad?" The rest of the visit my father recognized my brother. During that visit we even played a few holes of golf. Granted, my father was not able to play much, but he enjoyed riding around the cart with his son. These are the moments and the memories I cherish to this day. That visit also gave my brother an opportunity to see for himself how my dad was doing physically and mentally.

The reason I share this story, which was the last time my brother saw my father before he died, is to point out the importance of coming together as a family, whenever possible, on behalf of whomever you are caring for. I was lucky that my brother and sister did trust me and were grateful for me taking on the responsibility of the primary secondary caregiver role for fifteen months. My aunt and uncle also frequently supported my efforts with thanks and comments that they thought I was doing a great job. I wasn't looking for kudos, but it sure helped to boost my spirits to get them. Most fortunate, in this situation, was that my sister was there at this critical time when I really needed her help. And, what a blessing that was for each of us. As my father's life was slipping away, she was the one who was there for him at the end.

A Turn for the Worse

I was already in Michigan when my father's condition worsened. After being discharged back to the skilled nursing facility, he was very quickly returned to the hospital. Sadly, my father's swallowing issues were not getting better. I was called by the care team, who suggested that a "swallow test" be completed by the speech and language therapist. The test performed was a radiograph of his throat and lungs. The diagnostic benefit of this method was that they would be able to observe what happened while he swallowed different foods and different consistencies of food under diagnostic observation. The findings were not positive and pointed to many deficiencies.

The physician in charge of my father's care called me with a recommendation that was very upsetting to my sister and me. He recommended that a feeding tube be surgically inserted in my father so that he could be given nutrition, without having to eat orally. I had a very long discussion over the phone with the doctor to try to weigh the pros and cons of the feeding tube. He was adamant that this was the best choice, but also said that it was his opinion and that this was a permanent measure so once it was inserted into my father's stomach, where liquid would be poured in for nourishment by the nurses, it could not be removed without a court order.

Quality of Life

What came next was the most difficult decision that I had ever faced. Not being in Florida made it all that more difficult. The good news was that my sister was there at "ground zero," to be there for my parents and keep an eye on my father's care. I asked the doctor to hold off on a feeding tube until I spoke to my family. In the meantime, I did my research and spoke to each person working with my father and in particular those who knew him best.

My most important conversation was one I had initiated by calling the speech and language therapist, who had been working with him primarily to assist his eating and to make adjustments to how he ate and what he ate. He was eligible for this continuation of therapeutic service upon discharge from the hospital. However, once his progress plateaued, or in other words, no further improvement was noted, such services would discontinue. In this case, the progress stopped quickly. His choking had become more frequent and life threatening, despite feeding only pureed foods and thickened liquids. He had to sit at a special table in the nursing home dining room and was still separated from my mother.

After talking to my sister I called the speech therapist who did my father's swallow test and talked to her for about forty five minutes regarding my father's prognosis. I wondered how the feeding tube would help him. Would he get better? Why do this at this point in his life? Would he tolerate having a tube surgically inserted? What were the risks? I asked her, would my father ever be able to eat normally again? She answered, "No." This was a real blow for me to hear. Would it feel uncomfortable for him to eat by mouth? She told me it was a risk and no longer a pleasurable way to ingest food. I pursued some more questioning with her and because of her compassionate tone and willingness to listen and answer every question I came up with, I took the risk and asked her, "If it were your father what would you do? Would you have a feeding tube inserted?"

She answered, "No, I would not."

What was explained to me was that even with a feeding tube, when a patient has the amount of difficulty with swallowing that my father had, he would be at risk for pneumonia and choking even from saliva. This was surprising to me, so I did ask more than one person if this was the case. Off the record, many people who worked in the skilled nursing home section, as well as those who knew my father upstairs, were not in favor of feeding tube insertion. There were patients who had been fed via tubes for years, who had no quality of life and no hope for improvement or change. They simply lived life in bed with someone feeding them by pouring canned nutrition through a tube day in and day out, many without any family ever coming to see them.

I do not profess to suggest that you should make the decision that we did, because every individual case is different, and you may also have philosophical or religious reasons to make a different decision than we did, which of course should be respected. In our case, we had Advanced Directives and a Living Will. My sister and I had Power of Attorney and were his Health Care Surrogates, which my father had agreed to and had signed when he was of sound mind and body and he did indicate that he was not in favor of such measures to keep him alive artificially.

Hospice Care or Feeding Tube?

My father was sent out to the hospital for IV fluids to help stabilize him. The push was to insert the tube and send him back to the facility. The other option presented was to have hospice come in to do an assessment, to see if with his current presenting symptoms, and based upon his history, if he would be appropriate for hospice care. We found out very quickly that yes he was eligible. This was my first experience with hospice, so I read what they gave me very carefully. I then talked to my sister and to the person who did the assessment, to bring myself to a place where I felt secure in making this decision.

With my sister on site to observe and speak to my father, while I made important phone calls, we both gathered as much information as possible to make the biggest decision either of us had ever had to face. My sister also shared the feeding tube recommendation with my mother, who was not in favor of this option. My father's understanding of this choice was that he wanted to be able to eat to live, as my sister recently explained to me. At the same time, my sister watched my father trying to rip out his IV's and saw his lack of cooperation with the hospital staff. She questioned his care staff and they all reported that he didn't understand that the tubes and IV's were there to help him. All he wanted was to have a meal, and my sister told me that he thought they were starving him. His dementia and uncontrolled diabetes was a bad mixture and caused many problems at the end of his life. All we wanted for my father was peace and no more suffering at this point.

Because my father was at high risk for pulling his tube out should one be inserted, my sister asked what would happen if/when my father were to pull out his tube. The answer given her was that they would reinsert the tube and have my father restrained so that he could not pull it out again. And I found out, that once the tube is inserted, it could not be removed without a court order. Wow, this was a really hard decision. Ironically, my mother had the same condition as my father at the end of her life. Little did I know that seven years later, we would have to make this same decision again?

We, of course, contacted my brother and my father's sister, and they both agreed to call in Hospice, and to start what is called, "Palliative Care." This seemed like the best choice all things considered. Palliative care is a medical and multidisciplinary approach for providing the best quality of life and comfort care when near death.

Hospice and palliative care is something that came up in all four of my later caregiving experiences, but this was my first "rodeo," and it was definitely the most difficult ride in many ways. Making this kind of life-and-death decision is really very difficult at so many different levels. I was lucky in this case, because my sister and other family members agreed that calling in hospice was the best course of action to take. All professionals and family members, whom my sister and I consulted, thought that hospice was the best choice considering all of the variables including my father's prognosis. Only the facility doctor, who stood to gain financially by keeping my father alive through the use of a "peg" feeding tube, felt that hospice was not the best choice. I suppose he may have had religious reasons for his position, but considering he had quite a few patients in the nursing home on feeding tubes, who seemed to have no quality of life, I had a jaded view of his reasoning.

Hospice Care

If you never have had the need for hospice care for anyone, be it family or friend, then you may not have a full understanding of what this type of care involves and how it works. I know that I thought that I knew what this service provided, but when I actually needed it I found that I had a rather limited view of what it had to offer.

My father was allowed to die with dignity and even have the chance to have an ice cream milkshake in his final days. This seemed to relieve his feeling and perception that he was being starved to death, because the medical protocol was to discontinue feeding someone when they were unable to eat or drink without aspiration and choking. He was unable to grasp why he could not have food. He was nourished with small amounts of liquid, and had someone there to place warm compresses on his forehead and massage his hands and feet, if that's what he wanted. He was comfortable, and someone sat with him the entire final days of his life.

Over the fifteen years since my father's death, hospice has evolved into areas providing more and more assistance. My father's experience with hospice was different than my later experiences with each of my four other family members. To me a very significant benefit of hospice care was that it gave my family members the ability to die without pain and with dignity. I can attest to the fact that hospice was a Godsend in each of my experiences with my family at the end of their lives. Yes, each time was different and the needs different as well, but as a family member and caregiver, I found hospice care and the personnel involved to be extremely helpful most of the time.

I must add, that like anything, not all hospice agencies are created equally. For some reason, this didn't occur to me and I remember feeling so angry and frustrated when the service that I expected and was told would happen, did not happen, or it was done poorly by someone who seemed to lack understanding of what my family member needed, or they were overwhelmed and not there when needed. This I found out the hard way, fortunately on only two occasions, and it didn't include everyone in the agency, but was a significantly negative experience for me each time. I remember thinking, as if it isn't hard enough that my loved one is critically ill and near death, I am dealing with someone who is detached and giving me the run around, possibly not fit for the job, burned out or just not accessible when needed the most. No matter the reason, I learned to follow my gut when someone wasn't doing what I thought needed to be done for my family member and if necessary, I reached out to the social worker on the team or the supervisor to make them aware of the shortcomings of the person providing care.

The Final Days

Once my father was under hospice care, he died within approximately thirty-six hours of the paperwork being signed by my sister and myself. I knew that my father's death was imminent but did not believe that he would go as quickly as he did.

My sister had been with him praying the night before which was something that as a minister in training she felt so comfortable doing. She felt good doing it and she told me that my father really appreciated it. During her last evening with him, he told her that his parents were there with him, which is something that often happens near the end stage before death. While my sister was with my father he told stories about his life. He also entertained the hospice nurse by telling her his life story. He had a boost of energy and talked all night long with the hospice nurse and my sister. This burst of energy can and does happen when death is near. This may be hard to believe but I later learned that often people have a point of lucidity and energy before they pass and later witnessed it myself.

My sister was with my father most of the night according to her report to me but she also went upstairs to my mother's apartment to check in with her and be there for her as well. My sister had offered to take her downstairs to see my father, but she opted not to see him in his final hours to say goodbye. Of course, my sister respected her wishes and I agreed that this was best. I truly believe that my parents had been saying their goodbyes for quite some time. My mother wanted to remember him as he had been, not as he was. This is a personal preference, not to be judged by others. Each one of us handles death differently, and that's okay. Ultimately, my sister missed being at my father's side when he took his final breath sometime in the early morning hours. She had just left to go back to check on our mom. She prayed with him and comforted him in his final hours, which I truly appreciated and I am certain my dad did, too!

My Reactions

Not being there myself, did not come without my own feelings. I received the dreaded phone call from my sister while I was making breakfast. My sister's words were simply, "He's gone." I was crippled with grief and began crying uncontrollably in the laundry room of our cottage. I remember shutting the door and not wanting to see anyone. (I think we had company, but I am not positive of this memory). I could barely speak. I listened to my sister tell me the details of my father's passing and the hours before he left our world. Even though I knew he could die at any time, I honestly believed that he would not go so quickly. I could not believe what I had just heard, even though I knew he was dying. The pain of hearing that my father died cut through me like a knife. What strikes me is that intellectually I knew it was going to happen, and by all accounts it would happen quickly, but when I got the call, it was like getting struck by lightning. It felt so quick and it hurt so deeply that I could hardly catch my breath for quite a few minutes.

The one thing I took away most from the loss of my father was that I had very conflicted feelings about not being with him when he died. My sister and I talked about the fact that I had been assured by the medical staff that he wasn't near death. They told me that my father's heart was strong and that I had time to go to Michigan and come back. What I remember most, is that my dad seemed to rally whenever I came to see him. He would perk up for just a bit. I honestly feel that he might have been subconsciously protecting me from having to see him go. I found out over time that this is not unusual. Both my sister and I felt that this was true. We thought it interesting that he literally waited until I left the state before he "let go." She and I also felt that she was the one who needed to be there with him when he died. As I shared earlier, she had lost her husband so tragically and so instantly in the plane crash just three years prior, never being able to say goodbye him. Together we came to the realization that it seemed to happen the way that it did for a reason.

My need to get organized, and get back to Florida took me out of my shock, and I stepped into my action mode of getting things done. I needed to get down to Florida to be with my mother as fast as possible, giving my sister the chance to go back to Colorado where she had important commitments. I did what I had to do and flew back to Florida and made plans with the funeral home. I included my mother, knowing the importance of this. If she did not want to help or be a part of it, that was okay, too. I went with what she felt she could handle and I told her that I could do it alone if she did not feel up to accompanying me. My mother did not say too much, but was by my side as I spoke to the funeral home people. Fortunately, we had a pre-paid plan in place, so most of the decisions were in place. This is something everyone should do.

As I wrote this part of the story, I found myself recalling a few significant things. One, I do not recall my mother shedding a tear. She may have, but not in my presence. I also remember not knowing what to say at times and such times felt painfully awkward. My way to cope with this was to talk about anything but the memorial plans. My mother wasn't communicating, which was not unusual and part of the grief process. With her head injury, she had lost some ability with emotional expression. Yes, she was in the early stages of grieving, as was I, which is normal, but as I reached back in my memory to write this part of the story, I realized that we expressed our grief very differently. All of us did.

My sister and my brother also expressed their early grief in different ways that reflected, I believe, our basic personalities. My sister and I talked freely with one another and seemed to be in the take care of business mode. My brother and I talked more about feelings and he reflected on his memories of our father, as did I. And, over time, this changed as we moved further away from the initial shock of first experience of losing a parent. Yes, we all knew it was coming, but until it happens, we simply do not know how we will react.

Being analytically minded, I tend to try to understand such events in my life, and what I have learned most is that we cannot control these things, but we can accept what has happened and look for the positives of our experiences and cherish the good moments afterwards. I find that what I remember most about my time with my parents in Florida, were the good times we had when they lived nearby, and I was so comforted in knowing that they were safer being cared for in a way that none of us felt we could provide. Grief is something I have learned more about with each loss that I have experienced. Each time it hit me differently, which is not uncommon. I have gained new insight each and every time.

For my father, palliative and hospice care supported him at the end of his life. It gave him the opportunity to tell his life story to the hospice nurse and my sister, whom he talked to all night long two nights before he passed. It gave my sister time to pray with him and get support for herself from the hospice care staff.

My father went out doing what he loved. Talking to someone who would listen to his story, and have whatever he wanted to eat; no sugar restrictions, and no judgments made. One booklet that I was given from a hospice center in Michigan, which I will share in my brother's story, explains so much in a short and simple way, as to what we might see in the stages before someone dies. Reading this was very comforting, explaining so much about what I had already experienced at this point three other times.

Planning the Memorial Service

My father passed in June of 2001. He was cremated in Florida and I took his cremains back to Michigan with me where he would be buried in my mother's family plot. We planned a Memorial Service in the church where we summered in August, and figured out a way to bring my mother up for a three-week stay.

One thing that was immensely helpful is that we prepaid for his funeral arrangements in Florida and had made all of the decisions about cremation and urn selection before my father died. We had ordered ten death certificates, and all other things that go along with such details. I highly recommend that if feasible, go to a local funeral home to make arrangement and prepay, especially with elderly parents. In the long run money will be saved.

My sister and I looked at dates for my father's memorial service to be held where our family had summered dating back to my great grandparents in 1902. We decided that we would not bury my father in southeast Michigan, where there were already four plots purchased next to my father's parents, because my mother had told me during her last time on the island in 1999, that she'd prefer being buried in her family plot in Northern Michigan, not the one in Southeast Michigan. I said, "What about you and dad when the time comes?" Now, mind you this was about two months prior to my father's stroke in October of 1999. It was then that she said, "We both should be here!" I am glad I had the courage to ask this sensitive question. It ended up saving me the angst of making the decision without her blessings after my father died. I now knew where they wanted to be laid to rest. With my mother's decision, she also confirmed that she and my father should be cremated when the time came. You see, there was no more room in the family plot for caskets and there were only two spaces for two small urns left. Although not a lot of pre-planning was done, this issue was fortunately taken care of when I had the guts to ask my mother what her wishes were.

Moving Cremains Myself

Organizing the moving of my deceased father took on a whole new meaning. This trip meant taking my father's cremains in my suitcase when I flew from Florida back to Michigan. I finished the final details with the funeral home and saved some money by carrying his ashes with me on the plane. I remember my husband picking me up at the small airport in Northern Michigan and lifting my small bag and saying, "God, this is heavy! What's in this thing?" I answered, "My dad!" This is one of those moments where we laughed a little, but both felt the awkwardness of the moment. I was exhausted and grieving and wanted to get the trip over with as soon as possible.

Meeting with the Priest

As if the planning of my father's memorial service wasn't difficult enough, the day I went to talk to the priest in Northern Michigan regarding what we wanted for my father's memorial service, I was attacked by his dog, who was sitting on the front steps of his rectory. I am an animal lover and am not afraid of dogs. I walked into the white picket fence gate and closed it behind me and walked slowly up the walkway and looked into the eyes of this regal looking Gorden Setter. That's when the dog began his deep guttural growl at which point I decided to talk to the dog and tell him how beautiful he was. I looked into his beautiful brown eyes, which I now know was the wrong thing to do. The dog's growl suddenly changed to loud barking. I knew I was in trouble and I decided to try to turn away from him. As soon as I did this, the dog jumped up and aggressively leapt off the porch and attacked me. I was really scared so I swung my backpack at him to ward him off, but it didn't stop him from biting me in the rear end. Thankfully, I blocked some of his bite with the swinging of my backpack and I had jeans on which diminished the effects of the bite. Swinging my backpack gave me some time to get to the gate, but to add insult to injury, because of my state of panic, I couldn't get it to open to get away from the attacking dog. My hands were trembling and the thing was already tricky to get to open. The dog was still coming at me and barking ferociously.

People standing on the church steps across the street were watching this wild scene take place. At this point, I am pretty sure that I was screaming. That's when a clergyman came outside and called the dog off. He never apologized, nor really made any comment other than to call the dog and take him inside. I was quite rattled, but also relieved that my jeans protected me from his bite and my wound was merely a bruise. I recall thinking that it was bad enough to be planning my dad's memorial service, but to add insult to injury, the priest's dog had just bitten me.

Once the dog was secured I came back in for my meeting with the priest in his office. At my dismay, the dog sat on the other side of a baby gate and stared at me the entire meeting. I was distracted but managed to focus on the business of planning my father's memorial service, the first I had ever done. It was a memorable and challenging experience, and also a great learning opportunity. Thankfully, my family was there for me to ask their opinion and help. The important lesson for me was to make sure to coordinate with other family and, by all means, don't try to do it all yourself.

Saying Our Final Goodbyes

Two months after my father's passing, we held his memorial service in Michigan, where those who knew my parents best could attend, and family could come from near and far to celebrate my father's life. It was held in the Catholic Church and officiated by my sister, who was just recently ordained as a Methodist minister. She did a phenomenal job. I remember thinking about how she was able to hold her composure as she went through the service with poise and presence. My brother spoke about his relationship with my father extemporaneously and, in his way, charmed those who were there with his honesty and wit. He, too, held it together without breaking down or shedding a tear.

Now it was my turn. I had opted to write a poem and read it aloud. The poem was titled, "At Peace Now." My father loved poems and loved to write poetry, so this was my way of honoring him. Before reading the poem I shared that I had watched my father's mind and health decline and could see the suffering in his eyes and talked a bit about how hard the last few years of his life had been.

I started out reading the poem with strength and an unwavering voice, but when I got to the final stanza of the poem I cracked. I left the podium in tears, barely able to finish the last few words. Not unusual and not a bad thing at all. I do not regret having taken the risk to share what I wrote with those who cared enough for my father and our family to come to his memorial service. I also think that how I read the poem mirrored how I coped with my caregiving experience with him. I was strong on the outside from the beginning and fell apart at the end. The poem is on the back of the home-made program that my brother, sister and I collaborated on and produced the night before the service. I bought the paper and my brother did the graphics. And, as luck would have it, I found the program in a file with my father's death certificate around the same time that I was writing this part of his story. A coincidence; I don't think so. It was truly kismet to find it. Below is what I wrote and read in honor of my father.

At Peace Now

He's at peace now
No more struggle
No more sorrow
He's at peace now
Without pain
Without strain
He's at peace now
Ending his frustration
Ending his loss
He's at peace now
Minus the stress
Minus the agitation
He's at peace now
Free from restraint
Free from disease
He's at peace now
Leaving his legacy
Leaving his strength
He's at peace now
Remember his smile
Remember his love

Other Losses: This Was Different

I remember that after the service I was struck by how each one of us expressed our grief so differently; my sister spiritually and intellectually; my brother with his gift for entertaining and expression; and me through writing my feelings to convey that I wanted him to be remembered the way he was before his illness and dementia and that he was in a better place now. This is how I coped with my loss and deep feelings of grief.

What I learned from my experience with losing my father was something I never learned when I lost others in my life. I had lost all of my grandparents, pets, a twenty-one year old cousin and my brother-in-law, yet when I lost my father my grief was different. Loss is a part of life, and how we cope with it is the important thing to consider. I was fortunate to have my family to share my grief with, so that we could support one another in our time of loss. Not all families have this. I learned through my experience and through retrospection, that although grief is a universal condition, not everyone manifests it in the same ways, nor copes in the same manner. I think the key no matter what, is to find support in whatever way you feel comfortable. And, what I discovered with every loss I had after my father's death, is that I reacted differently. Yes, I grieved each time. The power of my feelings and the ways I coped also was different each time, because each relationship I had was different with the person who died. This may seem logical and expected, but honestly until I experienced it, I didn't truly understand it.

My caregiving did not end when my father passed. I, of course, continued to manage my mother's affairs, oversee her care and provide support to her in any way that I could, even if I was not nearby. For eight months we were still fifteen minutes away, but for four months I was in Michigan and she in Florida.

My role had been defined by the nature of my experience with both of my parents in what was now almost two years. I leave my father's story here and will now tell you about what it was like to help my mother in her final years. And, again, her health and cognitive issues were of utmost importance and I knew that even with the fact that she was living in an assisted living facility, I needed to remain connected, concerned and committed to helping her.

CHAPTER EIGHT

MY MOTHER'S STORY

During the seven years after my father's death I took care of the oversight of my mother's care. My experience with my mother over those seven years was in many ways the same as with my father, but also very different. As with anything in life, no two situations are alike. There may be similar situations, but the people, systems and other dynamics alter what happens during the caregiving experience as well as the outcomes of our involvement. In comparison with my father's experiences, some things in my role as helper with my mother were easier because of what I learned while helping my father. Other things were more difficult because I never dealt with a situation like it before, because the system I was working with presented new challenges or because of the differences in the personalities involved. What I learned from my first experience certainly helped me navigate my next experience, but it did not fully prepare me for all that was to come.

Following my father's death, we were all counting our blessings that my mother could remain in the assisted living apartment where she and my father lived for eighteen months. She had adjusted to the lifestyle and was comfortable there. An added benefit was that for eight months of the year, I lived within twenty minutes of her, so I could still be a big part of my mother's daily life. This is when our relationship began to evolve into something very special; something I wouldn't trade for anything, despite how difficult it was.

Staff Comments and Predictions

Soon after my father passed, some staff members working in the facility where my parents had lived, mentioned to me that it was highly likely that my mother would die shortly after my father's passing. This is often the case in long-term relationships. And, at the time of my father's death, my parents had been married just short of fifty-four years.

I imagine that for many people the staff's comments might be very upsetting. For my family and me it was not surprising. We anticipated that her health would deteriorate even further, and that she would feel lost without our father by her side. If you recall, she had already survived polio in her early thirties and a serious closed head injury in her early sixties. The closed head injury created a situation where my mother became quite dependent upon my father due to her limitations in memory. She was very bright, so she covered up her difficulties in many ways, and if you didn't know her before the accident, you may miss the fact that her affect was very flat compared to before, that she was not as engaged and forgot many things. And as she aged, she needed more and more help from my father. He was pretty much in charge of everything in their lives. Bottom line is that we figured she'd be lost without him.

My mother was a survivor. Throughout her lifetime, she overcame some very difficult challenges. Of course, I knew my mother from a daughter's perspective. When I stepped into the role as her secondary caregiver, things changed for me. I learned much more about my mother, as well as myself in this new role. I learned what I could handle and what I couldn't; what I was willing to do and not do and what I was afraid of doing. Over time, being my mother's caregiver gave me a newfound respect for her; one of the many benefits of my opportunity to be with her during this challenging time of her life. Surprising to all of us, my mother lived seven more years after my father died. They were not easy years, as there were many trips to the hospital and the need for much more personal assistance; however, with connection with family, stimulation from activities, the interest of old friends and proper care, she did far better than I would have anticipated and what studies and statistics and the facility staff would have predicted. She was fortunate to have the means to have good care and to have family who cared about her well-being. As we all know, this is not always the case. I contend that without caregivers, the statistics would be far worse.

My Mother's New Life Begins

The flight back to Florida with my mother did not go well. Our first flight should have been an easy connector but the plane had a mechanical problem so we had to take a van to a city two hours south without a meal and with my exhausted mother, who had just buried her husband. By the time we got a room, it was midnight and we had to fly out the next morning at around

6:30 a.m. for our connector in Detroit. A long van ride in the dark, a strange motel room, and a flight delay of one day was not at all what I had planned. Once again, I was faced with the challenge of not being able to control what was happening. It was especially challenging, but also an opportunity for me to grow and become more flexible and accepting of things I could not change or control. A pretty important life lesson for sure.

After a long forty-eight hours, we made it and my mother was back in her assisted living apartment, this time without my father. I was returning to Michigan the next day. Thankfully, she knew the staff and they knew her, so she had support and care. Still I knew this was not going to be an easy time for her. I returned to my home in Michigan a day after dropping her off, feeling sad, a bit guilty and emotionally and physically drained. Unfortunately, my trip back to Michigan was filled with drama, much like our trip back to Florida. I knew that I would be back to Florida in approximately two or three weeks but still felt bad about leaving my mother behind.

The date of my return flight was on September 9, 2001. My flight out of Florida was delayed, which meant my connection in Michigan was going to be very close. When we landed, I was directed to the gate I needed to get to and also found out I had only ten minutes to get there. To make matters worse it was very far away. I ran as fast as I could through the airport. The distance was about a mile from one end of this part of the airport to the gate I needed to reach. What seemed funny afterwards, but not as it was happening, as I ran frantically through the airport, I heard someone yelling behind me and when I looked back I saw my clothing was literally falling out of my backpack. I ran back and picked up what ended up being my underwear and resumed my run. I was breathless as I reached the gate of my connector, only to find the door shut. At this time, small jets like the one I was taking, were still accessed via the tarmac, not via a jet way. I pleaded with the gate attendant to let me on the plane. They thankfully called the pilot and asked him to wait, which he agreed to do. I ran down the steps to the jet and ran up the steps of the jet. I sat down exhausted not realizing what lay ahead the next day.

Amazingly, I made it home that evening and was able to sleep in my own bed. The next morning I was utterly exhausted and was taking it easy, drinking coffee and watching the morning news. The phone rang and I remember that I didn't feel like talking and almost didn't answer. Instead

I decided to answer thinking it might be someone calling about my mother. On the other end of the line was my aunt (my mother's brother's wife) calling to make sure I had reached home safely, and to see how my mother was doing after her long trip back to FL. I shared with her the difficulties of our trip and my own hassle on the way back up the day before. Ironically, as I was complaining about the fact that I almost missed my flight, I saw on the TV, which was on mute, the Twin Towers in New York City being struck by a plane. I was stunned by what I saw. On the other end of the line, I heard my uncle tell my aunt what he just saw on the news, which was exactly what I was seeing. We hung up so that we could figure out what was actually happening.

Like so many others, I remember watching in dismay and horror as the dreadful events unfolded of the now infamous day forever referred to as 9/11. I immediately realized when it was ordered that all flights be grounded due to the terrorist attacks that were occurring, I would have been stranded in Michigan. As I sat there and tried to process what I was seeing and hearing, what struck me most was the triviality of my own flight woes both down to Florida with my mother and my near-missed flight back to Michigan. I was so thankful that instead of being stranded in Detroit, I counted my blessings that I was let on the plane and that my flight was on 9/10/01, not 9/11/01. Those two days of travel are etched in my mind.

This was the beginning of many more future flights to care for family and it was a humbling experience to say the least. The series of events put a lot of things into perspective for me, as it did for millions of people that day. I lost my father and my mother was a new widow, but the tragic loss of so many innocent people that day dwarfed my problems and made me realize I was blessed.

I drove back to Florida shortly after this experience with my husband and the cats and everything went smoothly. Upon arriving back in Florida I immediately began my daily visits with my mother along with lunch one to two times a week. Things seemed to be going very well. She seemed to be adjusting to her routine and life without my father as well as could be expected.

My Second "Call" to Action

In early November of 2001, just six months after my father's death, and two months after the burial of my father, I made a routine phone call to my mother to say good morning and to check on her. The day before this pivotal phone call I had taken her to lunch at her favorite deli. When I picked her up that day, I recall having a gut feeling that she was a little off, but I couldn't put my finger on what I was seeing or feeling. She was quieter than normal and had complained about her right leg not working as we walked to my car. This is something I understand now that I should have paid more attention to right away. My own internal resistance to seeing anything wrong, along with my underlying denial, most definitely got in the way of my asking more questions and/or taking proactive steps to get help.

In retrospect, I should have taken her back inside to the nurse to have her checked before going onto lunch. Instead, I helped her get to my car and we went to eat. She wasn't hungry and she appeared vacant and disinterested. I was aware of the fact that something was not right, but could not accept it. It was my inner voice saying, oh no not again!! I was not ready for what was happening right before me. Having just lost my father, I could not accept that my mother had something wrong with her. I was like the ostrich with my head planted firmly in the ground. Or, the proverbial, "See no evil, hear no evil, and speak no evil" monkey. I just was not emotionally ready to accept what was right there in front of me. My mother and I did manage to get through lunch. I honestly do not recall if I mentioned any of this to the nurse on duty when I took her home after our lunch. I left my mother in her assisted living apartment and went home.

The Next Day

As I stepped into the shower the next morning, I had this strong feeling to call my mother right away. I jumped out of the shower, quickly dried and called her from the bathroom. What happened next was surprising at one level, but at the same time something I expected at a subconscious level. I started out with my typical, "Hi Mom it's me." I could hear that the phone had been answered by my mother as I could hear the TV in the background, yet she did not say a word.

I said, "Mom, are you there?" With a delay in reply and with a different sound to her voice, she answered, "Yes!"

"What are you watching on TV?" I asked.

She replied, very slowly and with a slight slur, "Julia Childs!"

Oh God, I thought, what's wrong? My immediate thought was that she was having a stroke! I tried to illicit some more answers but there was silence on the other end of the line. She was not responding to open ended easy questions.

I said, "Are you okay, mom?"

Her answer, "No."

I told her that I was going to call the nurse to check on her, which I did immediately. The nurse went to her apartment right away to take her vitals and call 911. She called me back right away and told me that an ambulance had been called and that I should go to Emergency room at the nearby hospital to meet her.

Once at the ER I found my mother alone on a gurney looking wide-eyed and very frightened. She reached her left hand out to me, and opened her mouth and nothing came out. I was so worried and felt helpless as we waited for what seemed like an eternity in the emergency room for the CT scan results. I had bought a newspaper and she reached to look at it so I gave her the section she enjoyed the most. She would pick it up with one hand, look at it, and then immediately set it back down. She did this repeatedly for the hours we waited for the results of the CT scan. It was a very long wait, with me talking and her just looking at me with distress in her eyes, while reaching for the newspaper and setting it back down over and over again.

I did try to read to her, but she was not following along and appeared detached, which was reflected in her facial expression. What saddened me most is that what I was seeing reminded me of what happened to my mother's expressiveness in 1985 from the bike accident. She had actually gotten better over the years. She was never the same, but certainly more herself. Either that or I had become accustomed to how she was. Nonetheless, that day her eyes had a look of fear in them, which for me was very difficult to see. Her repetitive attempts to speak without result, was beyond unsettling. I wanted so badly to make everything all better for her, but I couldn't. I felt helpless as I sat there waiting for the "verdict" on the CT scan. Nobody could offer any explanation as to what was happening. My patience was running out.

Finally, after what felt like an eternity, someone came to us to tell me that my mother had suffered a stroke and that she would first require hospitalization to stabilize, observe and assess her. First she was admitted to a general hospital room. After a few days of observation, the recommendation was that she be moved to another floor dedicated to therapeutic rehabilitation.

My mother spent five long weeks on the rehabilitation floor in the hospital. Her expressive speech was gone, unless she was asked simple questions that could be answered with one word. Her receptive language was still good. Watching my mother, someone who had an incredible command of the English language and a very large vocabulary, suddenly be unable to express basic wants and needs, was devastating and so hard to believe and accept. Yes, she had the earlier closed head injury in 1985, but she had adapted and her speech had not been affected in any significant way. Her short-term memory was poor, but she could carry on a conversation. No, not as well as before the head injury, but certainly far better than what I was witnessing now. I was scared and very sad. As with my father, I wanted to do everything I could to support her and anything I could do to make things better.

New Experiences and New Learning Opportunities

The after-effects of my mother's stroke affected the opposite side of her body from where my father's had been afflicted. The first difference was that my mother's brain was damaged on the left frontal lobe and my father's was the on right frontal lobe, both of which will cause different deficits and concerns. The side where the brain is injured from any trauma will affect the opposite side of the body. Unlike my father, who had "Left Neglect," my mother's stroke resulted in very flat affect, little facial expression, limited verbalizations and an inability to use her right hand as before. My father could walk just fine, yet my mother walked with an awkward unsteady gait with very poor balance, requiring assistance. This factor made a big difference in the amount of care required. She was not at risk in the same ways as my father. My mother's was her high fall risk and inability to get to a bathroom without assistance and some mental challenges.

One of the most difficult issues surrounding my mother's situation for me was rooted in the guilt I carried with me for not acting sooner, when I saw but didn't respond to, when my mother's symptoms first appeared the day we went to lunch. We all make mistakes and our own emotions can certainly cloud our vision. I could not change what happened, but what I could do is take what I learned and be more aware in the future and also maybe help someone else by sharing this story and acknowledging my mistakes.

Evaluations, Rehabilitation and Visitations

Just like my father, before my mother went into rehabilitation she was evaluated by a neurologist. My experience with my father's neurologist was very positive; however the doctor who saw my mother was a big disappointment. He was very gruff and flippant. As the neurologist evaluated her and asked questions, my mother slowly lifted her hand and pointed to the doctor's name tag. My mother then opened her mouth and struggled to say the doctor's name. It was painful to watch, but encouraging to see as well. My mother's way of communicating had evolved into pointing more than verbalizing. She pointed to buttons on my shorts as if to comment on how they looked. I became a pretty good interpreter as time went on.

My father's neurologist was empathetic and very forthright about what to expect: my mother's neurologist seemed to be in a big hurry and was dismissive towards me. The one major benefit of what he did was to explain and demonstrate to me that, with my mother's type of brain injury and communication deficits, she would be better able to speak by putting a phone in her hand. I still am not sure of the principle behind this, but it worked. Although I found out over time that his suggestion was very helpful, I could not shake the feelings I had with how he treated my mother and me during this initial evaluation. I felt compelled to let someone know, not to "tell on him," but to provide feedback so that perhaps another person and their family would not be put through an experience like I had. I think if I hadn't had the great experience I had with my father's neurologist, I would not have understood the difference and would have considered it as being normal and acceptable. I do recall making a formal complaint to the Patient Care Services department.

I bring this up to share the importance of advocating in a proactive positive way for your family member, especially if they for some reason or another cannot communicate for themselves. I felt the need to protect the next person who might encounter this doctor and his dismissive approach. In talking to the complaint department, I learned that this doctor was not employed by the hospital but had privileges there, so they could make note of my complaint but there was no internal review process. I recall feeling exasperated when I hung up, but at the same time I felt better simply telling someone about what had happened. Perhaps it would improve his bedside manner and the way he treated his future patients and families. Every hospital has a department such as this, but it may not have the same name. Such information should be in the materials given to you upon admission.

Visitations

Visiting my mother in the hospital every day became a routine part of my life. Hospital visits were made easier by the fact that I lived five minutes from the hospital in Florida and I would be there until June of the following year, so right away I knew that I could be there every day to support her. I went each day around 4:00 p.m. and stayed for her dinner in her room. Thankfully, the food was wonderful and she had a good appetite. We would call my brother or sister, so she could hear their voices and their news and also give her the opportunity to practice her own speech. We also called my aunt each day. It proved to be true that the phone was the best means for her to communicate and it certainly kept her connected to others who could encourage her every day. My mother always loved talking on the phone, something I've inherited, so this was a natural way for her to communicate. An added benefit was that I felt support from the process as well, and it made me feel connected and less alone.

Left Unattended

While my mother was in the rehabilitation section of the hospital for five weeks, I made sure that I made time in my day to oversee that she was being cared for correctly. Unfortunately, I oftentimes found her unattended to and left to lie in soiled diapers rather than taken to the toilet, where she could manage to go with some assistance. The rehab floor was maxed out to capacity, with patients waiting for beds. The nursing staff was insufficient for the demand, so my presence was necessary and vital to her receiving proper attention and care. With my mother's inability to speak for herself and her difficulty finding the right words to express her needs, she needed an advocate by her side whenever possible. She also needed some time to redevelop her independence by my not speaking for her all of the time. It's a balance that we would find together over time.

It helped that I was there often so those taking care of my mother knew that there was someone who cared for her who would be there to support her. I felt very responsible and wanted to make sure that she was cared for in all of the best ways possible. In order to do this, I realized from my experiences with my dad that I had to make sure that I was also supported. Supporters of others need and deserve support themselves.

Time For myself

Okay, so what could I do about my feelings? Ignoring them was not a good idea. Honoring them in some way seemed possible to me. What I learned was that I needed to make some time for myself and take breaks. Some of my breaks were during the visits themselves. If I was feeling tired, stressed or angry, I took walks through the hospital or went to the cafeteria for coffee or a bite to eat. Being there for my mother in her time of need felt like a duty to me. I didn't resent it, but I felt obligated. It honestly was not fun to visit and, in fact, was frustrating and upsetting. My mother's inability to communicate, as well as her inability to get to the bathroom without assistance, was not easy for me to take. The staffing was not sufficient for her needs, so I worried about her when nobody was there to watch over her. I knew that I needed to be there for her, and loved her, but honestly I had a difficult time sitting there day in and day out. That's one reason that I tried to go at mealtimes. It was a time when we could talk about things and "break bread" together. Oftentimes, she shared food with me and since I knew she couldn't finish everything on her plate, I accepted her offers to eat her food. Knowing that my mother would thrive with visits from me motivated me to be there for her.

To allay some of my concerns, when I was not there, I made it a point to call my mother and the nurse on duty to see how she was doing during the day. I called after morning rounds, in the afternoon and before the evening shift left to get a report. I am a firm believer in not worrying about bothering those who are caring for our loved ones. As good as hospitals can be, they are oftentimes understaffed. I needed to stay on top of her care and remain present in some way every day.

For example, because my mother could not adequately convey or verbally express her wants and needs I found, more than a few times, that people thought that she also could not understand what was being said to her or around her and so ignored her. From this experience, I have learned that if someone thinks that the person they are caring for cannot report anything to anyone, their care may be jeopardized when family or friends are absent.

Of course, this is not the case for all professional caregivers in hospitals, nursing homes, and rehab centers but it is not unusual.

CHAPTER NINE

TRANSITIONING FROM ONE LEVEL OF CARE TO ANOTHER

Five weeks after my mother suffered her stroke she was ready to be discharged from the hospital's rehabilitation inpatient program, but this did not mean that she was ready to go back to her assisted living apartment. As with my father, my mother was returning to a place that provided all three levels of care; independent living, assisted living and skilled nursing care within the same building. This meant that my mother went back to what was familiar to her. She wasn't ready to go to her third floor apartment yet, but instead was admitted to the first floor of the skilled nursing center. She could continue to receive physical, occupational and speech and language therapy. Because she had already bonded with many of the staff, especially the nursing supervisor on her assisted living floor, she was greeted by those who knew and cared about her upon her return. And, by those who knew my father as well, as this is where he had passed away approximately 8 months before. An added therapeutic benefit was that she was able to visit her cat in her apartment with my help when I visited. The transition was also made easier by the fact that there was a familiarity to where she was returning, which had become "home" to her.

What I learned from my time with my father, helped me to navigate the systems better, and gave me a new perspective on what I should be doing to support my mother. In addition, my mother's personality was actually easier for me to deal with, as she was not so difficult and combative. She was compliant, a "good patient." Staff saw her as easy to care for, which is a good thing in most ways. The flip side was I worried about her more because she couldn't report things that were not going well to others such as staff, or myself. This worried me greatly so I found myself being present to oversee her care as much as possible, which meant my life was once again on hold. I

93

am not complaining but I am explaining that I was willing to give up some of my time to be there for my mother in her time of need.

In the beginning of her therapy at the skilled nursing center, I was so hopeful that she would make great progress, speak again and be able to write, read and walk independently, but this wish never did come true. She was now more dependent than at any other time in her adult life. I tried to explain what was happening to my family, but until you spent time with her, it was difficult for others to grasp.

Upon discharge from the hospital, rehabilitative therapy was to continue on an outpatient basis to help her with basic daily living skills, self-care, walking and learning to adapt to the loss of normal use of her right hand, which she could no longer control or manipulate as she needed to or had been able to do prior to the stroke. For example, her hand would raise up without any intention on her part to do anything with it; when she wanted to pick something up like a fork, she could not control it. Her dexterity was also poor. She could not write like she used to nor draw as she had before. The plan was for her to continue in therapy in the skilled nursing but because she "plateaued" in her progress rather quickly, it was discontinued.

Medicare as with most insurance covers post hospitalization out-patient therapy. In my mother's case she continued therapy in the skilled nursing section of her assisted living facility, until she showed no more evidence of improvement. Medicare does requalify patients for further therapy after a period of time has elapsed, in hopes that progress can be made again later on in the healing process. After six weeks, reapplication for more therapy can be initiated and prescribed by the primary care physician. New learning can take place, and the brain can often develop new pathways to supplant areas that were damaged by a stroke or other brain injury. This requalifying happened for my mother about every six weeks, but then she would "plateau" again and therapy would discontinue.

There were other benefits being at the skilled nursing center. She most loved anything musically oriented and what turned out to be great were sing along times put on by the Activity Director. A life-long music lover, with a great memory for lyrics, the staff were delighted to tell me that any song that my mother knew from her past she could sing along with, knowing every single word. The Activities Director in the facility was so pleased to tell me of how she loved coming to hear musicians play and always smiled and laughed and seemed to truly enjoy herself. This is the kind of thing that helps to stimulate healing (release endorphins, the happy hormones) in the brain. I remember coming to join her during these times and just watching her have some fun again gave me so much joy and hope myself.

Other activities were not as fun for her and she would tell me in no uncertain terms when I asked her. For example, they had bingo a few days a week and I would ask her how she liked that and she'd always say, "I hate it." Nonetheless, she would be compliant and play, and I know it was helpful for her to do, but I got a kick out of her honesty. She would slowly get the words out, and would turn and look me in the eyes whenever she told me she did not like something. My point here is that, it was important for her to have the opportunity to participate in things, and yes, if she really didn't want to do something they didn't force her. However, stimulating the brain via different activities makes a difference in improving functioning. At her age and with her history, the gains were not as great as someone younger, but any gain was worth the experience.

A Need for More Supervision

The challenge for me as her caregiver was the fact that my mother needed more oversight than what the assisted living provided. For my mother to be discharged from the nursing home, we had to figure out the best way to provide an added safety net. At the same time, she qualified for less than what skilled nursing could provide. I learned that our best option was to hire a part-time private nurses' aide to stay with her during times when she needed assistance to bathroom. She had no way to call for assistance from an aide on duty on her floor, other than to pull a cord, which was already in the bathroom or by her bed. We wanted her to be able to sit in her medical electric recliner in her living room, where she could keep her feet elevated for circulation and where she could see her TV, her window to the world. This was her favorite pastime now that she was no longer able to read books as a result of the stroke.

My mother was not able to safely use her walker consistently, even though we placed signs all over her apartment that said, "Use Your Walker." Her short-term memory was very poor and made this modification inconsistently helpful at best. My sister and I now joke that they should teach kids in preschool how to use walkers so that when and/or if they need to use one later in life and their ability to learn is poor, they will have learned it at a young age, which would be "old memory." As baby boomers continue to age and live longer, I see a market for the next generations to get ahead of this problem with early life practice and training in some way shape or form. Food for thought anyway.

To help, we hired a part-time aide. The process of hiring a part-time aide turned out to be easy, in that they were already available within the facility, which is not always the case. Through word of mouth, I was able to line up someone to be with my mom during times of transition, and/or times that she would need help with bathing, as this proved to be the most difficult situation for her. We hoped that having someone there with her midday, a time when there was not sufficient staffing, would help to prevent falling and loneliness. I could come most days by 4:00 or 5:00 p.m., and the aide typically came from 11:00 a.m. to 3:00 pm.

It was a huge relief knowing someone was there for my mother. Grief over the passing of my father was still fresh, so I knew my mother must be lonely, along with her significant physical and cognitive limitations. Under these circumstances, I felt very fortunate to be in a position to hire someone to fill in the gaps. Thanks to real estate sales, she was able to afford the benefit of extra assistance. This gave me a sense of security and I felt like things were under control, so I felt it would be okay for me to head north to Michigan as I had been doing.

All Seemed Good For Awhile

For quite some time, things went smoothly. The aide was pleasant and my mother enjoyed having company and help. All seemed good and it gave me a sense of comfort, while also permitting me to do the work I wanted to do with the county school system and a children's charity and work on another children's book. I also was able to play the sports I enjoyed, which was very important to my physical and mental well-being. I am a person who needs physical activity; that's how I relax. When I was doing long daily hospital visits, without exercising the way that helps me, and without eating right, my own health was at risk and in fact was impacted.

My mother actually was happy that I was carrying on a long family tradition. She liked to hear about everything going on where she and my father had spent years visiting together. Sharing my experiences helped her to access her own special memories. Knowing this, I checked in every day by telephone with my mother and the private duty aide.

Another Call

Things went well until September 2002, when this time I received a call from the nursing supervisor for the assisted living floor and she told me that my mother had fallen in the bathroom and was being transported by ambulance to the hospital. I was back in Michigan at the time. The nurse suspected that she had broken her hip. The time of day I received this call was during the time that the aide should have been there in the apartment with her. I immediately began asking questions and quickly learned that the aide "did not feel well and went home." The aide had left mid-shift and assumed my mother would stay right where she had last sat her down, which was in her motorized reclining chair that we had bought for her comfort and to assist with getting up out of the chair. The fact that the aide did not let me know that she was leaving early infuriated me. If I had known, I would have called the supervisor to see if someone else could check on my mother.

I understood that the aide was ill and could not stay, but I was very angry about the fact that she didn't tell me she had left early. The world is not a perfect place, I know. And, accidents and mistakes happen, but in this case I felt that what had happened was negligent on the part of the aide. No, I never took legal action, but I did not hire her again.

So how was it that my mother was found on the floor in her bathroom unable to get up? Well, thanks to my cousin's suggestion, my mother had gotten a medical alert system installed before I had headed north for the summer.

My cousin's suggestion to get something like a medical alert system came from a discussion she and I had following my mother's stroke, based upon my concerns about her overall adjustment to her new life without my dad, along with her new physical and communication limitations. We talked about the fact that she could not remember to pull the emergency alert cord on the wall by her bed and in the bathroom if she needed help. In addition I was concerned that if she fell where she couldn't reach the emergency cord, then what? I knew about medical alert systems, but didn't think about getting it because I figured my mother had a built-in "safety net" where she was living. I think that had I been on the outside looking in, I probably would have thought of this great idea myself. My own high level of emotional involvement clouded my judgment.

Fortunately, the way my cousin presented this idea to me was not pushy and was done in such a way as to not come across as critical. I have found that sometimes when we're in these situations, we feel so overly responsible for everything, that we can miss the bigger picture, and thus may be unable to realize alternative solutions. This is why talking with others is so important. Reaching out and sharing concerns, oftentimes leads to good ideas. It's not that I was stupid not to think of this myself, it's more the case that the closer we all are to someone, the more difficult it is to, "see the forest through the trees." In my case, I was overwhelmed and was trying to think of everything. At some level I wanted to believe that everything was taken care of by the facility I had found for my parents.

Amazingly, when my mother fell in the bathroom that fateful day, she did remember to push the button on her medical alert system just like we had practiced (and as the company had recommended). And sure enough, when the medical alert company answered the call, a voice came over the speaker in her bedroom and asked her, "What is your emergency?"

I asked her, "What did you say when they answered your call button?" She told me she said, "I've fallen and I can't get up!" This was amazing to me and a testimony to the power of commercials. And, it made me laugh, giving me some humor that at this point was needed. Being a TV watcher she probably heard that phrase many, many times and thank God she had. It worked like a charm and the ambulance was sent and the facility was notified of the emergency in her apartment, so the nurse could go sit with her until help arrived.

Flying Back To Florida

When I received the call that my mom had fallen and probably fractured her hip, I knew right away that I would need to get on a plane ASAP and go to Florida to help her. I was dreading the trip. The usual anxiety about all that went into the logistics of travel at a moment's notice, the strong feeling that I wanted to stay home in my comfort zone with my husband, my cats and my routine, welled up inside of me. I wish I could say that I was able to "go with the flow," but honestly, I may have looked like I was taking things in stride on the outside, but inside my stomach was churning, my breathing vacillated from holding my breath to rapid breathing. I felt consumed with uncertainty and just wanted to be able to control more of what was happening in my life. I was able to "get a grip" after the initial shock that my mother was injured, despite the safety precautions put in place.

Long distance caregiving had become something I dreaded. The unpredictability of the travel and the cancellation of things I wanted to do or had planned sometimes bred contempt. The flip side of these feelings was the strong guilt I would feel for having such feelings. And, at this point, I had not figured out how to release these feelings in healthy ways. I knew it would help to find someone to talk to, because honestly, my husband was not the right person at this point. He took care of things for me when I was gone, but he wasn't too keen about rehashing my trip experiences when I returned home and needed to debrief.

My sister was often the one I would call, and that didn't always go well either. Our talks would start out well, but I found myself feeling defensive when she would offer advice or suggestions. We were too close and had our established sibling issues. My sister was extremely busy with her new life endeavors, so I tried not to complain too much, but I needed somewhere to vent, so I am sure I wasn't always cheery and optimistic when we would talk.

In this case, although I knew I should get to my mother fast, I had no way to make this happen quickly. Luckily my dear cousin had already planned to fly down to visit my mother for the weekend and because of this, she was able to be there during my mother's hip surgery. I then would arrive the following day after she left to return to work.

Having my cousin as another support system was an incredible bonus. She loved my mother and was ready, willing and able to help. I was learning that I could trust others who offered to help and I learned that I could stay connected to the professionals providing my mother the medical care and support she needed. Trust for me was a big issue, as were the deep feelings of guilt when I couldn't be there when I felt that I should be the one to oversee things. Becoming more accepting of help and letting go of some control was a big step and a recurring theme for me throughout all of my caregiving experiences.

Safety and Health Concerns

I was able to get down to be with my mom after my cousin left. While healing from the hip surgery, my mother developed a sore on her leg that was extremely painful. I noticed it on her shin area and asked a nurse about it. It turned out to be "cellulitis." In my mother's case it was considered to be the result of her surgery. In addition to the fears I had for my mother's safety, the other most difficult thing with this situation was the tremendous pain my mother experienced; a very hard thing to watch.

It is a helpless feeling when you cannot relieve someone else's pain. With my mother's inability to express her needs, this became a bigger concern for me. This was my first introduction to being with someone who was basically helpless and in excruciating pain. To add to this, my mother was unable to remember how to summon for help, i.e. ring her bell for the nurse. On top of this, when someone did come to help her, she had difficulty telling them what her need or problem was. When she did try to speak, it took time and it was very frustrating for her, and for those taking care of her as well. For some staff members providing care for my mother, waiting for my mother to get her words out was a problem. I saw it as a lack of patience and understanding and it worried me to say the least. I tried to understand their perspective and their own time constraints and the very fact that they had more than just my mother to care for. However, my logical/intellectual brain was oftentimes overcome by my emotionally overwrought brain. Day in and day out of looking into my mother's eyes and seeing her own fear and frustration took its toll.

My challenge was that realistically I knew that I could not stay there for any extended period of time to be my mother's "watchdog." I also knew that once she was released to go back upstairs to her apartment that my mother clearly needed someone to assist her more than just a part of the day. As a high fall risk and someone with expressive speech deficits she definitely needed more oversight. I immediately began asking people who they might recommend to help keep her safe when she was alone in her apartment. I asked the Supervisor of nursing if she knew of anyone and was quickly relieved to learn that one of the most admired and dedicated aides in the building had just become available due to the fact that the man she had taken care of for twelve years had just died and she was looking for someone new to help with daily needs. The misfortune of one family became our families' Godsend.

I immediately sought her out to see if she would be interested in caring for my mom during the most high-risk times in her day, and/or when she required extra assistance. This aide said that she would, "love to help my mother," and she already knew both my parents. She offered her condolences for the loss of my father and had kind things to say about him and my mother. She seemed genuine and compassionate. I hired her right on the spot. She ended up being with my mom until the day she died. My mother loved her and felt safe with her; she was our families' angel on earth. We were blessed by the care and companionship she gave my mother. We all loved her! She and I still stay in touch.

As my mother's needs grew, the aide's time expanded to twelve-hour day shifts. She recommended a friend of hers to take the night shift. The night shift nurse was not nearly as good or reliable, but seemed to be perfect until we unfortunately found out the hard way that the oversight during the night was lacking, which led to an accident, that to this day, I believe could have been prevented. However, no matter what prevention safety net you have in place to keep those you are caring for safe from harm's way, accidents can and do happen.

This time, my mother was injured when the aide tried to keep her from falling while coming out of the shower. The aide, in an attempt to assist, grabbed my mother's arm, causing a shoulder injury. This accident was most likely the result of a poor transfer technique. Nonetheless, it meant she required an x-ray, and more care, including more therapy. This led to her spending time in the skilled nursing center downstairs again. The upside of therapy as I saw it, was that it gave her more opportunities for social interaction with others and there were professional caregivers observing her, which increased the amount of individual care and support she received. It increased my mother's opportunity to engage in verbal interaction, even if the helper was doing most of the talking, it included asking her questions that she needed to answer. There are pros and cons to everything and in this case, the con was the injury in and of itself, but the pros in my mind outweighed any negative aspects of the therapy experience.

The Psychologist

In addition to physical, speech and occupational therapy, my mother received psychological support for depression and this I saw as a very important aspect for her overall well-being. I knew that she was grieving over the loss of my father, her husband, as well as her own diminishing abilities, which was normal, but as her daughter, I was not able to provide the type of support she needed in every way, so I requested an assessment and the psychologist was in agreement and was a great fit for my mother. This was a relief to me to have someone other than me for my mother to confide in. I really liked her therapist, which was great. If I thought there were a problem, I also knew that I could file a formal request for consideration for a change in personnel. This fortunately was not an issue at all.

I share this because I had a very difficult time when my efforts to help my mother somehow fell short. With emotional distance from such events and my experiences has come some wisdom. I understand that I could only control so much and that my efforts were what mattered most. I put things in place with the intent to protect and make my mother's life as comfortable as possible and that was what was important. My feeling like a failure or worrying about everything all the time was not productive, nor healthy. This is not to say that my personality didn't lead me to repeat this tendency in future caregiving experiences, but awareness of my proclivity to obsess over what went wrong did help me to be more self-forgiving when things I could not control all the time happened with negative consequences.

Changes, Losses and Decisions

A few months prior to moving my mother downstairs, her cat "Winnie" died. It was a very sad day. I knew it was coming and had asked the aide to please tell me when Winnie stopped jumping up onto the sink to drink water from the kitchen tap as she always had. She did not call to tell me this, as she did not want me to have Winnie euthanized. This decline in the cat's behavior and health was normal as she was about twenty-two years old. I tell this story because it was another loss, for myself, my mother, the aide, the assisted living floor and my family.

Anyway, my nephew and his wife had just come in from Wyoming for a visit. I took them to see my mother. When we arrived at her apartment, I saw the cat lying under a table. I went to her and found she was very ill and I knew then that it was time to take her to the vets to have her put down. The "kids" looked at me with sadness in their eyes, both being big cat lovers, and watched me as I gently wrapped the cat in a towel and put her in the soft sided airline carrier we brought her to Florida in and placed her in my mother's lap and said to her, "Do you want to say anything to Winnie before I take her to the vets"? She replied slowly and deliberately, "Nice knowing you!"

This comic relief was very welcome, especially for my nephew and wife. They could not help but giggle a bit and looked at me and waved as I left to go to the vets. She went quickly and without pain. I remember being more broken up than my mother. This was because of her loss of ability to express emotions. I fortunately understood this and had no expectation that she should have behaved differently and certainly didn't say anything critical to her about her response to the loss of her cat. For my nephew and wife, it was surprising; however, they "got it." Her emotional distance could be attributed to her change in sensory awareness and blunted emotional connection from her stroke.

The loss of the cat was the end of an era. She was the pet my parents got to be a companion for my mother after she had her head injury. Turned out my father really bonded with the cat more than my mother, because he needed her more at the time and her head injury blunted her ability to connect emotionally. And, really, my mother didn't pay any attention to her after her stroke except to look at her and point at her occasionally, but she was still very important to her.

The Cost of Care: More Decisions

Despite good financial planning, the cost of my mother's care depleted her savings six years after my father died. At about the same time she required more care than could be provided in Assisted Living, due to increasing health and safety issues. I cannot recall the exact timeline here, but do remember that we made the decision to let the night aide go, and we moved my mother downstairs into Skilled Nursing full- time.

This process was an experience in and of itself. The day I told the aide that I would need to let her go did not go smoothly at all. I explained that I would give her two weeks' notice and that I would come see her that evening when she arrived at work. My mother was there in her wheel chair waiting to go to dinner and the night aide was very angry and disrespectful toward me.

I asked her to come out in the hall with me to talk and she said, "Why, she (meaning my mother) doesn't know what we're saying!"

My mother said, "Oh yes I do!!!" I will never forget that for as long as I live. The words were minimal, but they spoke volumes. Any doubts I had about letting this aide go were allayed immediately. My mother was a woman of few words after her stroke, but when she spoke, it was always meaningful. A lot could be packed into three or four word utterances.

We retained the daytime aide and continued to pay her ourselves with some help from other family, such as my cousin. Again, her communication issues were of most concern and she could not remember how to call for help. Most importantly, her relationship with her aide and now friend, Juliette, was of utmost importance. For me, knowing that she was there for my mother during the day was a blessing to say the least. She got a shower every day, and had a companion as well. She helped her to answer family phone calls by picking up the phone and handing it to her. Support like this meant that my mother could stay connected, not just to me, but to my sister, my aunt and my brother.

Applying for Medicaid Assistance

My mother's health needs were now exceeding what the assisted living apartment could provide her, plus the expense of the aide was a big factor as well. My mother's funds were quickly depleted once we had to move her into the nursing home downstairs for long-term residential care. Our only choice was to apply for Medicaid. The process of applying for Medicaid was difficult, confusing, depersonalizing and more challenging than I had ever imagined. Even with my educational background and training as a social worker, the hurdles that had to be jumped to complete all of the paper work and to ultimately produce all that was required to be eligible for Medicaid insurance was an intimidating and sometimes exhausting process. It took organizational skills, perseverance and above all patience and an ability to wait a long time on hold. The year was 2007, so I cannot speak to the process today with the new healthcare law, but I would venture to say from what I have read and heard, the process continues to be difficult. My point here is that it makes sense to me why so many people have gone uninsured; the process is extremely cumbersome.

One particular moment in the process that I recall vividly was the first time I had to walk into the Department of Social Services office in Broward County Florida. The attendants were behind glass. The first person I approached would not look up when I walked up to the window. I knocked softly on the window to get her attention. She barely opened it a crack, gave me instructions and some paperwork to fill out and was rude and dismissive. Because of the glass and the fact that she mumbled and spoke softly, I could not understand what she was saying. I asked a few questions and still needed more specifics, so I asked if there was someone else that I could speak to and she nodded and after I sat in the waiting room completing the form, I was invited in to a room to speak to a caseworker.

I found out what I needed to gather for proof that my mother's bank account was below $2,000 and that she did not own any property and had sold her homes before the three year "look back rule." This was the timeline in place at the time. I honestly don't know what the rules are at this time, but know you can find information online. The difficulty of the process is compounded by all that it represents. I tell this part of my mother's story, to underscore that as a caregiver, you may be faced with things you are not prepared for and this factor makes it all that more difficult. Given this, the importance of being brave enough to advocate for those you care for is of utmost importance. What I found is that these experiences taught me the difference between assertiveness and being pushy and demanding. A good lesson indeed.

I was successful in getting my mother Medicaid, which paid for her long-term nursing home care. This was a good thing, just not easy to achieve. I found myself spending countless hours pulling it altogether, which meant less time for me. I did not resent it. I just think it's worth pointing out the reality of things.

Moving Again

I feel it's important to point out that when I had to move my mother again from her assisted living apartment to a semi-private room in the nursing home downstairs, it meant sifting through the things we had almost eight years before brought down to Florida that were particularly sentimental to my parents. Another "radioactive" event for me.

Thankfully, my sister came to help me move my mother's things out of her assisted living apartment and once again had a more pragmatic approach to the process. Going through some of the same things that we had already moved from my parents' Michigan home made me realize how hard it is to let go of memories held in objects. When I first packed up my parents' most valued treasures and photos and sent them to Florida ahead of their arrival, I put photos, art work, and personal accolades in a small closet in their apartment.

At some point in this process, my brother came to Florida to see my mother as well. He weighed in on things he wanted to take with him. I remember one particular item he took with him one night, which was a damaged painting that always hung in our foyer of our childhood home. It was a portrait painting of a young man who we were told was "Uncle Henry" from five generations back. He took it home one night, saying he would ship it back to his place in Michigan. About an hour later he phoned to tell me that he threw the painting out in a dumpster in a parking lot on the way home. This is the kind of struggle that can happen while making decisions about what to keep, throw out, sell or donate.

Having my brother there for part of the moving process was especially good for my mother and his presence gave me a break and also gave my mother much joy. She would beam with delight each time he came to see her. I was there the most, so my being there was routine. He was her only son, need I say more.

I won't go into all the moving details. Suffice it to say that with each of my five experiences as a caregiver, moving other people and their valued possessions proved to be one of the most challenging aspects of my role. Each time I faced this "job" I got better at throwing things away, organizing the process and delegating and asking for help from others. Moving symbolized the end as well as impending loss and sorrow.

CHAPTER TEN

THE FINAL MONTHS: DEJA VU ALL OVER AGAIN

It became apparent that my mother was beginning to experience difficulty with eating because of swallowing difficulties. Her appetite was good but the food would not go down properly causing coughing and choking reactions. To me it seemed unbelievable that it was determined that my mother faced the exact same problem with eating and swallowing as my father had in his last few months of his life. I remember thinking that maybe because they had been so close for so long, that they even ended up having the same problem. What I later discovered is that dysphasia, as I wrote about in my father's story, is a common concern in nursing home settings and it is often associated with strokes and dementia as well as the aging process.

Like my father, her difficulties were treated with a change in diet and assistance while she ate. There were also attempts to teach those who helped her learn how to feed her to reduce aspiration and choking. I remember feeling devastated that I had to witness another parent choke when they ate. I was struck with such sadness when I learned this news. However, unlike my father, my mother was far more cooperative and accepting of help. On the other hand, I cringed when I saw her look of distress and attempts to pull away as helpers spoon-fed her.

Those caring for my mother felt it was their duty to do everything they could to get her to eat. My mother was a pleaser so with a second attempt of encouragement by her aide, she would eat. I felt physically ill as I watched my mother being force fed by hand and grappled with what was the "right" thing to do. I decided that it was best to seek the advice of her primary care physician in the facility. I told the nursing supervisor that I wanted to see him when he next came in to check patients. By this time, I also knew what day he came and made sure that I was there when he made his rounds so that I could catch him to ask him questions about my mother's condition and care.

At this point in my life, my only experience with end-of-life eating difficulties was with my father and if you recall that was not easy. Ironically, my mother had the same condition as my father at the end of her life. Little did I know that seven years later, we would have to make this same decision again. As with my father, one option to consider to help my mother was to have a feeding tube inserted. Sound familiar? My mother's doctor had a different perspective and opinion about feeding tubes than my father's doctor did seven years prior. I told my mother's doctor of my earlier experience with my father and what we did for him. This doctor agreed that a feeding tube was a choice but not the optimum one for my mother. Instead hospice was suggested, and I was very relieved. The doctor also suggested that my mother not be forced fed. If she didn't want to eat or drink that was okay. He assured me that she would not feel thirst, hunger, or discomfort.

Advanced Directives

It was my "job" to talk to my mother to explain why she was having so much difficulty with chewing, swallowing food and drinking fluids without choking and to explain what options were in front of us as to how to best help her at this point. Thankfully, my brother was down for a visit and I thought it would be good to have him there for moral support for me, and my mother. He listened but did not interrupt as I took time to explain clearly and slowly where things were with my mother's current condition. I opted not to involve the doctor at this point, but did reference him by telling her that I had spoken to her doctor and asked what measures could be done to help her. I also invited my mother's aide to sit in and listen as well. If we came to a place where the medical doctor's explanation would help, I was very open to his assistance. I explained that we needed to look at what else could be done to help her. I added that she was at risk of pneumonia and choking. I reminded her of the tough decision we had with my father, which she remembered, or at least said that she did. Next, I read to my mother what she had previously signed with respect to her wishes in her Living Will and "Advanced Directives." I asked my mother whether or not she still felt comfortable with what she had signed and she said, "Yes" and when asked if she wanted to change anything, she said, "No."

This talk was not easy, but it was certainly necessary and I did so out of respect for my mother and to give me some peace of mind as well. My mother knew that she was facing the same thing that my father went through, and I thought she had the right to weigh in on this very important decision. In this case, although my mother couldn't independently verbally express her wishes, she was able to answer questions and was clearly aware of what the questions meant. As a result, I did not feel comfortable simply abiding by the more general words of the Living Will, so even though I was the assigned Patient Advocate/Healthcare Surrogate, with my sister listed as secondary, I felt it important to ask my mother what she wanted.

POLST and Advanced Directives

Years later, Advance Directives have advanced themselves to be more specific, as to what one really wants done to sustain or not sustain their life when the time comes for such very tough decisions. These are important documents, but the conversation about what people really want in respect to comfort care, hospice, life-saving/support measures, etcetera helps those left to make the tough decisions to understand the wishes of the person who such choices effect the most. POLST stands for: Physicians Orders for Life Sustaining Treatment. For more information you may visit websites such as www.polst.org/advance-careplanning/polst-directives.

"Having the Conversation"

While doing research for this book, I met a woman named Ronnie Genser, who based upon her own end-of-life experience with her husband, started a company called, Bereavement Navigators (www.bereavementnav-igators.com). She educates financial planners, attorneys, etc. on the subject of making final plans and the importance of having someone else's wishes spelled out ahead of time, which makes all the difference in the world. Unfortunately, this is oftentimes easier said than done.

Recently, Ronnie Genser, contacted me about an organized effort to educate and provide tools for people for such times through what they call, "Having the Conversation." The group is called the "Conversation Project" and can be found online at www.theconversationproject.org. I believe that much of the distress my family and I went through could have been avoided or at least lessened if we had a conversation far before any of this happened. Talking with our family about our wishes and being specific about them, not simply by signing a legal document, but by spelling out what we really want before situations occur where life sustaining measures must be evaluated and decided upon, be it a feeding tube, resuscitation, medications, intubation, and life support machines, definitely could have helped me in all five of my caregiving experiences.

Interestingly, I think most people would agree that this is a great idea and statistics support this notion, but actually having this conversation with our loved ones is a completely different thing. What I learned from my experience is that the conversation can feel and be uncomfortable. It is probably something most of us want to avoid; however, it could prevent situations like I faced.

Second Guessers

One way such conversations might help is when others, who also care about those we are caring for, have strong opinions and "second guess" the difficult end-of-life decisions we may have to make. What they may think is right or wrong when it comes to end-of-life decisions might be diametrically opposed to the wishes already expressed by the person whose life is on the line. In my case, when I tried to convey to my mother's aide what the doctor told me, and to explain that for my mother eating was no longer pleasurable and in fact painful, and could cause pneumonia and continued aspiration and choking, this conversation did not go well. It was a very stressful and uncomfortable exchange, because the aide felt that I was starving my mother.

To add fuel to the fire, while having this discussion another aide from the building and a friend to our aide, who we all knew and loved, came to the room to visit my mother. When she heard that hospice was being called in to help my mother and that the plan was to stop making my mother eat, she accused us of starving her. I had to ask her to come outside of the room with me and to not talk like this in front of my mother. I told her I understood her position, but felt it was not her place to interfere. We were going with the doctor's recommendations and my mother's wishes.

This was a very stressful situation and I assume is something others are faced with when decisions surrounding swallowing issues are concerned. Nurturing others with food is something that is important all through our lives. Food provides comfort, sustenance, social interaction and is not just nourishment, but is a ritual in our lives. Feeding someone who cannot feed themselves increases the significance of the relationship and what it means. We feed babies, but adults who can't feed themselves, due to health and mental problems, are different, in that the dependency complicates the decision to withdraw food.

What was hardest about this situation is that it is already so stressful to make the decision to bring in hospice and not provide "food," but when you add to it the "second guessing" from other family members or friends, it gnaws at your own decision. I learned that as caregivers, we need to have good information and do our research to feel as comfortable as possible with our decisions to help make the right end-of-life decisions. Every situation is different and deserves careful consideration of options.

Hospice Again

I would describe the last few months with my mother as being a time of bonding, forgiveness and acceptance of things that could not be changed. I would also say that the end of my mother's life was a time of healing for me. Yes, like my father, my mother's inability to eat was the ultimate cause of death. But unlike my father, she did not have the behavioral issues that my father had, which meant for me much less turmoil. My mother did last longer than expected, but I attribute that to her determination and desire to live.

Summer was approaching and I had to make a decision regarding staying in Florida with my mother, or staying with our normal schedule of going to Michigan the end of May. This is a schedule my mother kept and she liked the family tradition started by her great grandparents being continued. She liked to hear of the goings on with her friends and family and seemed okay with my leaving. I was assured that my mother was still strong, and I could leave and come back in a few weeks, just as I was told with my father. And, like my father, my mother was okay for a couple of weeks. I quizzed the hospice nurse as to whether or not she thought I should come back and she assured me that death was not imminent. Same thing I was told about my father.

This Time I Was There

As with my father seven years before, in the same month of June, while I was up in Michigan, thousands of miles from my mother, I got *the* call. The call came from the hospice care coordinating nurse; the same one who had told me a day or so before that there was no rush for me to come down yet. This time she told me to, "Come as soon as possible!"

Now, mind you, I had told the nurse approximately two days prior that I needed at least twenty-four hours' notice to get down to Florida. My Michigan home was remote and travel to and from took some logistical maneuvering. I literally received a call at approximately 11:00 a.m. on my cell phone and was told my mother had taken a turn for the worse. I was able to speak to her on the phone to tell her that I was on my way and would be there as fast as I could. She uttered something that I could not understand. I felt frantic, surprised and overwhelmed with the thought of racing off to be with her as she was dying. Mixed emotions flooded me. Thanks to my husband's support, I managed to pull it together.

I landed twenty-six hours later in Florida, with very little time to spare. The minute that I could turn on my cell phone upon landing, I called my mother to let her know I had made it to Florida and was on my way to be with her and that I loved her very much. The aide answered the phone and told my mother I was calling and held the phone to my mother's ear. I spoke to her and told her I would be to her room in about one hour. My mother was no longer able to respond to anyone and was being kept comfortable with morphine, warm compresses, and hand holding by the hospice team, which consisted of a nurse and social worker. Attempts to save her life were off the table due to clearly spelled out advanced directives. Hospice was in charge of her care with the nursing home support there if necessary.

Fortunately, the shuttle that I had pre-ordered was there waiting for me curbside and amazingly everything went like clock-work, and I made it to be with my mother before she took her final breath. I had called again once in route to let my mother's aide know that I was in route. She again held the phone to my mother's ear and I told her that I would be with her very soon. I heard labored breathing on the other end of the line. Having mixed feelings doesn't express the way I felt. On the one hand I wanted to get there quickly, but on the other hand, I wanted time to stand still.

One of the things I recall was that for some reason, even though it was midday, we had little traffic compared to a typical day and we made it without delay to my mother's facility.

When I walked through the nursing home doors, I was greeted with a hug from one of my mother's nurses. I was flooded with emotion. I recall being hugged and rushed along at the same time and told by more than one person as I jogged down the hall that my mother had "waited for me." I was struck by overwhelming emotion and also tremendous relief and enormous trepidation. This situation was the epitome of "approach-avoidance." I wanted to be there for my mother, but I was scared to see her in the condition she was in and during her final minutes on earth. Death is a natural part of life, but I had never been with anyone who had died before and I was scared and deeply sad to say the very least. I really didn't know what to expect.

I wanted her to be free of pain and suffering, but didn't want to lose her, even though she hadn't been the mother I had who could talk to me, walk with me, read books, and enjoy all the things she had before her stroke. At this point, who she had been was not what I was losing. I was losing my "mom," which also meant I would no longer have parents.

As I entered her room, the hospice social worker was there along with an array of staff members who loved my mother. I recall feeling smothered by their presence and what sounded like cackling voices. I needed and wanted to be alone with my "mom" but couldn't find the words to ask everyone to leave. The social worker sensitively and gently asked me if I wanted to be alone with my mother. I was so relieved that she took charge of the situation and asked people to leave me alone with my mother, which they all respected and left the room.

The loud voices were gone and now I was faced with saying goodbye to her for good. The social worker asked if I'd like for her to stay and I said, yes. I was scared and welcomed her quiet presence as she sat in a chair and occasionally made a supportive comment. I remember feeling safe and supported. I needed someone with me. Even though I knew professionally what to anticipate in terms of emotions, nothing could fully prepare me for what I was about to witness and experience. What I understood from what I had read in hospice information was that we need to let the person go and that may mean telling them that it's okay.

I remember feeling so helpless standing there stroking my mother and speaking to her about things that came to my mind. I wanted her to go peacefully, but it wasn't a smooth transition to watch at all. She was gasping for air, with her breaths becoming more and more irregular and difficult.

I told my mother that I would always miss her but that I didn't want her suffering any longer. I cried the entire time that I talked to my mother.

Also from my reading, I had learned that the last sense to go is hearing, so I was convinced my mother could hear my words of support, honor, love and acceptance for her to die. I was so much more emotional than I could ever have imagined that I would be. I was never much of a crier, so when I was so distraught I remember feeling out of control, even though I wasn't. What I was going through was all normal; nothing weird about it.

I sat down for a minute, and took a break and gave my mother a break as well. Within a minute or so of my silence, my mother stopped breathing, and the time of death was called. I was totally quiet, as was the nurse and the social worker. I then softly said, "She's gone!" With that utterance, my mother took another breath. I went to her side again and told her I would be okay and that she could go be with my father and those who had gone before her. I kissed her again and left the room to go to the restroom. I felt that she would not "go" with me in the room.

I was told that it didn't take long after I stepped out that my mother took her final breath. One of the nurses on staff met me as I was walking back to the room to hug and hold me and she told me that my mother had passed. I believe that her maternal love kept her going, and I know now that this is not unusual.

My mother died just ten days short of her eighty-fourth birthday. She was a strong woman, who overcame many hurdles in her life. I miss her sense of humor and way with words. We still quote the many clever sayings that she used. She wasn't perfect, of course, and our relationship was not always great, but with age comes wisdom and in this case love conquered all.

Welcome Support from Staff Members

After my mother died, I was approached by a few of the nurses who were especially close to my mother and that knew me from my daily visits and oversight of her care. To a person, everyone began by thanking me for letting my mother go and for not having a feeding tube inserted. Any self-doubt about the end of life decisions made was lifted by this support. It is important for me to say that this was an individual and personal family decision, as well as respect for my mother's wishes. Intellectually I was sure it was right, however, the emotional side of me questioned whether or not we did the right thing. Having the support of health care professionals who watch patients die day in and day out with different levels of support and advanced directives meant a great deal to me and helped me to feel confident in what we did. I have never "second guessed" our decision since. What this experience did for me in a positive way, stayed with me when I was faced with similar situations with my next three caregiving experiences.

Cremation, Travel and Planning

What I had learned from my experience with my father helped me with taking care of my mother's Memorial Service plans and funeral home arrangements, which included cremation of my mother and again the logistics of pulling everything together. It was easier this time as far as the "taking care of business" aspect; however, the feelings of loss and grief were not any easier. I had learned the ropes the first time with my father, but that didn't ease the pain.

My mother's ashes were to be shipped to the summer cottage where my family would be gathering for the memorial service. I was assured that they would arrive within two weeks. This did not happen. I was frantic when the day before the service my mother's ashes had not arrived.

My sister was cool, calm and collected and was not the least bit worried. I, on the other hand, was a wreck. My sister said not to worry, because we could have the graveside service without the cremains and it wouldn't matter. To me, it mattered a lot. I felt like I couldn't have closure with this hanging over my head. For my sister, being a minister, this was something that she had dealt with before and to her it wasn't a big problem. I took it as a failure on my part somehow and I was distressed. My control issues reared their ugly head again, which is typical during times of stress.

After many calls to the funeral home in Florida, thankfully, one hour prior to the service the cremains arrived. We stopped at the post office to pick them up on the way to the gravesite. This was another lesson in patience for me. I was told that Florida State law required that they held the cremains for a certain time period before sending them across state lines. I still don't know if this is true and at this point it doesn't matter, except to say that while you're making plans ahead of time and you have paid for everything years ahead, make sure you find out the details of shipping so that you know before you are under duress.

What we had planned for my mother's service was different from what we did for my father. For my mother we had a graveside service, officiated by the minister of the church, which I had joined after my father's death. Although my mother had never clearly spelled out what she wanted for her end of life wishes, other than that she wished to be cremated, I had a clear idea of what I wanted to have and ran my ideas by my sister and brother. One thing I asked was for my brother to play guitar and sing the song "There is a Season." It was perfect! It was a song that seemed very befitting and also one I am sure is played at many end of life celebrations. My sister said a prayer, which was beautiful.

I wrote and read a poem entitled "Always a Lady" at the graveside service in honor of my mother. The title and verses came from the words of people who had cared for her over the years in assisted living and in the nursing home. They would often tell me that my mother was, "Always a lady." They explained that my mother was polite and always said, "thank you," something they said they did not often hear. My mother had an air about her that myself and others saw even through her physical, cognitive and expressive language deficits. I unfortunately could not find the poem I wrote, but feel the title says it all.

We had a lunch reception at the same place we had my father's and had made posters with photos of my mother to display. This is not unique but the process of getting it ready with other family members and friends, was special and memorable.

The lesson I learned through my journey with my mother is that relationships can be strengthened during such times, or for some they can fall apart. I learned so much about my mother's determination and strength during this time in our lives together. I treasure these years tremendously. They were not easy, but certainly well worth it. By the end of my mother's life we were very close and I grew to understand her differently and appreciate her gifts and her strengths and that she was a good mother, not always the one I thought that I wanted, but a mother who I could love and respect and thank in the end. I am grateful to have had the opportunity to help her and be with her at the end of her life.

CHAPTER ELEVEN

EIGHTEEN MONTHS LATER: MY AUNT'S STORY

It was approximately eighteen months after my mother died, when once again a phone call led to my needing to step into the long distance caregiving role for family. This time it was my paternal aunt. I thought I had experienced plenty with my parents, but with my aunt my role as caregiver presented some different challenges. I was especially close to my aunt, my father's sister; the same aunt who was very supportive of me when I was helping my father and mother up in Michigan after his stroke in 1999.

To give you an idea of our closeness, she was the one who helped me with my wedding plans and was my confidante through much of my adult life. She had also been extremely important to my siblings and myself in our early years. She was an essential support to my parents when my mother had polio after I was born. She was the aunt with whom I would go spend the night and would spoil me with undivided attention and nurturing when I was young. I had nothing but good memories of her. She was not just my aunt: she was my friend, and a woman whom I admired greatly for all of her lifetime accomplishments. My aunt had no children, like me, something we shared in common. And, she often told me that I was like a daughter to her, which presented different feelings and challenges surrounding my role and responsibilities when I had to step in as her long distance caregiver.

No matter where I was living, near or far, my aunt and I stayed in touch by phone. I looked forward to our talks. We talked about family news, her health problems, my uncle, my parents, my job and other daily happenings. When cell phones came on the scene and I had a long commute to work, I would call her to pass the time on my drive. We talked about everything! I was the one who told her what was happening with my brother and sister and our nephews. Because I had lived near her when I was first married we would reminisce and talk about people we knew in common. I had worked for them one summer as well. I particularly enjoyed my aunt's family history stories. Although she told the same stories many times, I never stopped her from sharing them.

Most of my life my aunt was my sounding board. I appreciated her words of wisdom and liked hearing her voice. She was the person in my life who always encouraged and believed in me. Her own life success was an inspiration. We had a mutual admiration for one another and it was something I needed and appreciated.

My Aunt's Accomplishments

My aunt was a woman of many talents. She was a pioneer as a female from her era. She was the only woman in her Medical school back in the early 1940's. She told me the story countless times about the Dean calling her into his office and suggesting she get married and drop the idea of medical school, not because she couldn't cut it, but because it was a different time for women. Sadly, my aunt never was able to complete her schooling, due to a case of tuberculosis, causing her to drop out in her third year. She never returned to medical school, but after one full year of quarantine in her home, with her mother as her caregiver, followed by a very long recuperation period, she was able to land a job with a major oil company as a chemist. She traveled to New York City for a period of time in the 1950's.

She was a successful single woman in what was then, a man's world, until she met my uncle. While playing golf with a group of men, they suggested she meet an assistant pro they thought she would like. She ended up marrying him, even though she was twelve years older. I would later tease her by telling her that she was the original "cougar." I was six years old when she married and remember that day well. Shortly afterward, she moved out of state. I remember missing her terribly and looked forward to her visits at holidays and sometimes during the summers. The closeness we had was rekindled later in life after she and my uncle moved back to Michigan, and I lived nearby because of my husband's work.

I share this background, because my early history with my aunt, played a big part in how and why I ended up being a secondary caregiver to her and my uncle later in life. I want to show that despite all of her abilities and accomplishments, it didn't prevent what happened to her later in life. My aunt's intelligence, tenacity and strength helped her hide the difficulties that were going on in her life at home. She still seemed sharp when talking to anyone at the grocery store, where everyone knew and loved her; she was very friendly and treated people with respect. She liked her simple life at home and didn't need a busy social life anymore.

Much like my parents, my aunt gradually lost her ability to manage things as she had before. However, she hid it well, so no one knew that she was failing. Her decline led to a very unsafe situation. Dementia and some health problems are not always that recognizable in the beginning. It can take over quietly, behind closed doors and then one incident can change things forever. This was similar to my parents, yet the details are different.

Hidden Problems with Dire Results

The irony of my aunt's situation is that during our talks over the phone, she was especially critical of my parents for not accepting help for their needs. And with everything that I had gone through with my parents, the thought of my aunt being in a similar situation clouded my perception of their situation. Deep down I did not want to know how my aunt was really doing despite some pretty obvious clues. For example, my uncle occasionally answered the phone and alluded to the fact that my aunt was worse than I knew. He would say things like, "She's sick as a dog" or "She's really bad! She sounds good when she talks to you, but she is not good."

I was living in Florida and they were in Michigan, so all I could do was make suggestions to my uncle. I knew that my aunt was not open to any help, because she told me they didn't need any. My uncle vacuumed and did the laundry. He was now driving her everywhere because of her failing health. I believed he was still capable of helping her so I didn't push things. I felt that their life was under control; not perfect, but manageable and not yet at a critical level of need. I also figured that because my uncle was so much younger and still seemed okay, that my aunt was in good hands. I was wrong!

My aunt always loved cooking and made breakfast and dinner for my uncle. At some point, I learned that she was still putting together cereal in the morning. However, my uncle was going out for both lunch and dinner at a local diner and would bring food home to her. I later learned that she was not eating well; her appetite had declined due to her health issues and aging. My aunt also suffered from pancreatitis, crippling arthritis, and small fractures in her spine from osteoporosis, frequent illnesses and urinary tract infections. She would go to the doctor regularly; however, it became more of a social visit. She enjoyed the attention and the conversation with her doctor. Their relationship began when she was his first patient years before.

My aunt loved going to see this doctor, her "friend." She would pull herself together, put on a nice outfit, and with her NY Times puzzle in hand, go to her appointments. Initially she drove herself, but when her health was failing my uncle drove her. She often said that what he prescribed didn't help her, but come to find out later, this may have been because she never filled or took the prescriptions given to her. I also know that she would go home and crawl back into bed and watch TV for much of the time. I found out later that my uncle never set foot in the office according to her doctor. He sat in the parking lot. I am not sure he was ever invited in actually.

Even the doctor was fooled and thought my aunt was doing well in terms of her mind and ability to manage her life. I, too, did not realize the depth of their problems. I was about to learn much more about how bad things had become. My personal resistance to seeing, hearing and accepting what really was going on with my aunt was rooted in my recent experiences with my parents. Plus I was very far way. I honestly could not fathom dealing with what I had experienced with my parents. Basically, I did not want to know, what I did not know. I stayed in touch, and prayed that my uncle could continue to care for my aunt. They seemed to have a system that was working somewhat until my uncle's own health took a turn for the worse. At least that's what I thought.

A Change in My Uncle's Health: Aunt at Greater Risk

My uncle's ability to be my aunt's caregiver was compromised when he was diagnosed with diabetes during a visit to the emergency room. I don't know what symptoms drove him to go to the ER, but what I do remember is my aunt telling me my uncle's blood sugar was at a dangerously high level. This diagnosis was a turning point for their life in more ways than one; none of it was good.

My aunt, because of her time in medical school, felt that she could give my uncle his insulin shots and they could manage the situation themselves. The problem with this plan was that she had very severe arthritis in her hands, leaving her with very poor dexterity. She also had essential tremors. Her head and her hands shook all the time. This made it very hard for her to steady the needle for injection. In addition, her organizational skills were no longer very good. This is something that is an issue for many aging people in our society today. Inside many homes, medical needs are not properly met or managed. Health and safety is a major concern for many. My aunt could have received home health care, but to her this was out of the question. Neither one wanted people coming into their home.

The Day I Called

When I made a typical "check-in" phone call to talk to my aunt in October, 2009, I immediately knew by the weakened sound of her voice that something was wrong. Initially, I thought she was sick, which was more often the case than not at this point in her life. I sat nervously at the other end of the line wanting to know what was wrong. At the same time I was afraid of what my questions would reveal. Despite my apprehension, I began asking questions, the first one being, "Are you okay?"

The answer was, "Your uncle fell!"

My first source of information about what had happened to my uncle was from my aunt. She told me that my uncle had fallen and that he was not home! She thought that my uncle was at the hospital and that, Mike, the guy from the gas station had taken him there. She sounded a bit confused and wasn't speaking as articulately as in the past.

When I asked my aunt where and how my uncle fell, she said that she thought that he fell in the parking lot. My aunt was understandably shaken by what had happened and was confused about some of the details, such as when the fall actually happened. Furthermore, she didn't know what was wrong with him exactly. It seemed this had happened at some point the day before, but I could not be certain. At this point, what mattered most was for me to determine his injuries/condition and where he had been taken for treatment. My aunt's information was sketchy but of grave concern. There was just enough information to tell me that I had to take action quickly. Exactly what that action would be was unknown until I could gather more information.

Fortunately, because I had lived and worked in the area where they lived, I was familiar with the hospitals and was able to figure out where my uncle was taken for treatment. 911 was not called, and as with my father, it should have been. I didn't know how to reach "Mike" at this point so I called the hospital where I assumed my uncle most likely was taken and learned that my uncle had been admitted. Unfortunately, because I was not on any of the paperwork as someone they could disclose medical information I was unable to find out anything other than that he was a patient in the hospital.

I stayed in contact with my aunt throughout the day and was trying to determine if I needed to hop on a plane to help her. She kept telling me that he was coming home soon, but I could not be assured that this was accurate. She sounded weaker every time we spoke that day. I encouraged her to drink water or any fluid and to eat something. I had no idea how bad her own health was at this point, but knew that it was not great.

I went back and forth in my mind trying to decide what I should do next. I learned from helping my parents that it was sometimes easier to get information from the night shift people in the hospital or nursing homes. The floor was quieter and the staff seemed freer about sharing information. So, later that night, I got ahold of the nursing station on the floor where he had been admitted. I reached a nurse to whom I could ask specific questions. She listened as I told her my dilemma regarding needing to know just how serious my uncle's condition was to determine whether or not I needed to fly up to Michigan sooner rather than later.

Given the fact that there was nobody in the area that could come to the aid of my aunt and uncle, I pleaded with the nursing supervisor on duty to tell me the seriousness of his condition. I phrased my question as such: "Given what you know about my uncle's medical condition, and the fact that my eighty-nine year old aunt is alone in her condominium, without anyone there to help her, should I get on a plane as soon as possible to come up to Michigan?"

Her answer was, "Yes."

I was on a plane the next morning by 7:00 a.m. and landed in Detroit by 9:00 a.m.

When I called and told my aunt that I was on my way, she told me to first go see my uncle at the hospital, which I did. In retrospect, had I known then what I knew a few hours later, I probably would have opted to check on her first. Before I tell you what I found at my aunt's condo, I will tell you what I learned about my uncle.

Prior to my arriving at the hospital, I was able to call my uncle in his room, to tell him that I had flown up and was there to help my aunt and to come see him as well. He seemed quite disoriented and told me a story that did not make any sense at all. He knew who I was over the phone, but was clearly confused and was very worried about my aunt. I assured him that I would be going to help her after I first came to see him for a short visit.

Once I got to my uncle's hospital room, I was told that he fractured his back and also hit his head. He apparently was walking to his car and tripped on a curb. At this point in time, I had no advance directives and nobody was assigned to be my aunt and uncle's Power of Attorney. I knew that through my urging they had begun the process with a local attorney to get their affairs in order, which my uncle did do, but my aunt had never signed the paper work. She had a million and one excuses as to why she could never find the time to go sign their Last Will and Testament, Trust and Advanced Directives/Living Will. My uncle had signed this paperwork approximately one year prior. And, the only reason he had gone to have this done was because my husband and I encouraged them to do it because they had no children and no direct heirs. Fortunately, when my uncle became better oriented, he was able to tell me the name of the attorney and approximately where her office was located. Again, my familiarity with the area made this part much easier.

From what I remember, the hospital did not have anything available for me to sign, nor did the hospital facilitate a means for assignment of someone to oversee my uncle's needs if he was unable to do so. Since then, upon admission, much has improved in this area, so that patients can appoint someone to make decisions when they are incapable of doing so at the time for medical or other reasons. In this particular case, my uncle arrived at the hospital confused from the fall. I don't know some of the details surrounding the first two days but my guess is that my aunt may have been contacted; however, she was in no condition to help. To complicate matters, nobody in the hospital had an alternative number/person to call. If I had not made the call to check in with my aunt that day, if it wasn't part of my routine to check on them, I am not sure what would have happened to my aunt.

Worse Than I Ever Imagined

When I walked into my uncle's room, he was receiving bedside physical therapy. He had also been walking the hall with assistance with a walker and appeared to be very weak and unsteady. I learned he was under control and seemed more lucid than our prior conversation over the phone. He knew who I was and was anxious for me to check on my aunt. I talked to the nurse and learned that he would require long-term therapy and stabilization of his medical concerns and physical limitations and that going home was not going to happen anytime soon. Like my parents, upon discharge my uncle would need inpatient rehabilitation. With this information, I knew that my stay was not going to be quick. And, how much ability he would regain was still unknown at this point in time. My next stop was to drive to check on my aunt. My worries were increasing by the minute!

As I drove into the parking lot, every ounce of me was tense. When I walked into the condo, it was dusk and all of the lights were off. I called out my aunt's name but there was no response. I repeated her name loudly and frequently as I fumbled around to find a light switch. When I got the lights on, I walked toward her room while continuing to call out her name to no avail.

As I reached my aunt's bedroom at the end of the hall, it was dark, but with the hall light on I could see her curled up in the fetal position with no sign of movement and still no acknowledgement of my presence. I was afraid that she had died. With much trepidation I approached her and touched her shoulder and she finally moved and moaned. I was able to get her to answer some questions but she was extremely weak from dehydration and no food. I turned on the light next to her bed and did everything that I knew to get her to drink some water and eat something. I remember feeling so afraid and overwhelmed with what I knew I may be facing in the months ahead and I wasn't sure I was up to the task at this point. Like many people, I knew that this was not a choice; it was something I needed to do.

What to Do Next?

That night, I called my sister to tell her about what I had learned and found and told her that I would keep her posted. I also called my brother to alert him that I may need his help since he lived about two hours away. I helped my aunt call my uncle and she felt better talking to him and letting him know that I was there with her. I actually lay in bed with her and talked. I assured her that I would stay with her as long as necessary.

I was exhausted emotionally and physically, yet so wound up. My aunt wanted me to sleep in my uncle's bed, which was in the "office" right next to her room. When I entered the room to get organized and watch some TV what I found was very upsetting. There was blood on the floor and on the blanket and sheets. I felt nauseous thinking of sleeping in this room. I stripped the sheets and changed them and tried to get some rest, but too many thoughts were racing in my head and I could not get comfortable. The condo was in complete disarray.

I needed to formulate a plan of action, starting with deciding who to call first. As luck would have it I actually had my aunt's doctor's personal phone number in my contacts in my cell phone from a time when he gave it to me in case I needed his help. I had met him a few summers back when my aunt had told him to call me to meet him and his family in Michigan when they were vacationing. This turned out to be quite fortunate.

I reached her doctor right away and we spoke for about an hour about what had happened and my aunt. Most importantly, I explained the situation regarding my uncle's fall and the condition of their home and my aunt's inability to care for herself alone. I asked for his help in encouraging her to either accept assistance in her home or go into a care facility to build up her health and strength while my uncle was rehabilitating. By telling her doctor ahead of her appointment, it gave him the necessary heads up for him to support my goals to do what was best for my aunt. It also gave me a chance to see what other options there may be based upon his medical opinion after he examined her.

The doctor admitted being surprised by what I had found in my aunt's apartment and was shocked at how bad things had become. He really cared for her and told me she had been his first patient when he opened his practice. I heard in his voice that it was difficult for him to accept what I was sharing with him. I emphasized that she could not be alone and that she did not want help in her home, which meant that she needed placement in an assisted living facility. What I needed from him was support in my efforts to keep her safe. He offered to make time for my aunt the next morning and told me to come in around 10:00 a.m. to examine her and also help me talk to her about the need to be somewhere where she would be cared for while my uncle was getting better. In this case, my aunt's friendly relationship with her doctor paid off.

When I hung up the phone, I was relieved to have the appointment set and tried to relax but couldn't. I had changed the sheets but there was only one blanket to use and it had blood stains on it, which I had a hard time dealing with. I still couldn't get the sight of the bloody sheets that I had seen earlier out of my mind as I closed my eyes. I had a fitful night's sleep, but felt good about being right next to my aunt's room in case she needed me. She was doing much better after I helped her to drink and eat a little bit, but I knew that she had other health concerns, one being very irregular blood pressure with spikes of very high to very low. I peeked my head into my aunt's room and checked on her about four or five times that night. In addition, my cat's aunt, who meant the world to her and my uncle, was in need of food and water. I immediately realized I needed to figure out what to do about "Inky," too!

What occurred to me rather quickly was that my role as supportive niece was instantly upgraded to caregiver, which meant that I had to take over my aunt and uncle's affairs. I am sorry to say that I honestly did not want to step into this role, but knew that there was nobody else who could help them at this point in time; not because I was so special, but because I was the person who could do it right then and there. I was overwhelmed by the thought of going through many of the same things that I had faced with my parents and, quite frankly, I wanted to run for the hills. I could have opted not to help, but because of the position I was in it would have been a very selfish choice on my part. I do understand that for some people, the option to do this would not be a viable choice.

I recall a friend of mine asking why I had gone to help my aunt and uncle and questioned me as to why someone else couldn't do it. I felt very defensive and tried to explain my position, but realized the person could not relate at all to my situation or feelings. The phone call left me questioning myself on the one hand, yet on the other hand, it made me feel more committed to doing what I thought was the right thing under the circumstances. In retrospect I still believe I made the right choice.

"Caregiver" isn't just a title one is given; it is a commitment that must be taken seriously and with forethought. I could have blamed them for the predicament that they were in, but knew that would not be constructive at all. Dementia, as I discussed earlier, does not look the same with every person. My point in sharing this exchange, is that second guessers often made me doubt my choices. In the long run, I learned to stay the course of what I felt was best for my family members in need. I also learned to listen to others when their input was constructive, not judgmental.

A Plan of Action

Thoughts of what to do spun around in my head all night long. By morning I had a plan of action with priorities in place. I knew that my aunt could not stay in her condo alone and the amount of time that I could stay was limited. With my mother, I stayed a full five weeks in the beginning, and I knew that this time I could not make such a commitment and hoped that I had other options available to me. First step was figuring out just what those options were.

Below is the short list of what I needed to attend to in order to put things in motion.

1. Call my uncle
2. Take my aunt to her doctor's the next morning
3. Locate someone local to be my personal backup whom my aunt could trust
4. Call my aunt's church for support
5. Locate and contact the attorney
6. Research alternative living arrangements

Completing these meant non-stop management. Making plans and taking action reduced some of my feelings of panic and stress. I wish I could say that things always went smoothly, but they did not. My first action was to take my aunt to see her doctor.

The Doctor Visit

The next morning my aunt was very weak, making it difficult for her to get dressed and get ready to go to the doctor. I made her breakfast and brought it to her in bed. With help and much encouragement, I managed to get her to get out of bed. Believe me, this was no easy task. She required full assistance with getting dressed and showering. She insisted on showering alone, but I helped her in and out and stood by for safety precautions. Her room was a mess, which was so unusual for her. Her clothing was dirty. I was able to find some items in the closet for her to wear that were clean and gave her some choices. When it was time to leave, she put up some resistance, but I just kept pushing the importance of her seeing her doctor, that he was counting on seeing her and had set aside a special time for her.

By the time we got to the doctor's office she was more alert, and as I described earlier was able to pull herself together to see her favorite doctor and friend. But she was still so visibly weak. The doctor explained to my aunt that she was weak from infection, and that her blood pressure was extremely high. Come to find out, she was missing doses and doubling doses of her blood pressure medication, which led to wild swings of blood pressure. He gave my aunt a new prescription that she proceeded to take incorrectly, which plummeted her blood pressure while I was staying with her, so I began keeping track for her. It scared me to think of how often this happened. The sooner I could find a place for my aunt to go for safety and support the better.

Fortunately, her doctor agreed with me and supported my goal to place my aunt in a safer assisted living environment, something I was now very familiar with. He told her that he thought it best that she not be home alone and that she consider what I was saying. I hoped that this would help her accept the idea. I had found a place to tour that had a respite care option and thought I could sell the idea better if it was seen as a short-term option until my uncle was well enough to come home. My aunt listened to me, as I told her that her meals would be prepared and she would not have to worry about shopping, or cleaning and that she could get stronger with help. She would say it sounded like a good idea one minute and then say things like, "Your uncle would not want me to go anywhere!"

What the doctor said to support my concerns had gone in one ear and out the other. This situation reminded me of my parents trying to help my grandmother when I was about thirteen years old. I recall stories of my grandmother firing every home health support sent to help her as she was not safe staying alone when my grandfather went to work. She ended up burning her arm severely when she passed out and fell on the radiator. She had sent the helper away, "fired her," and my parents did not know this.

Sadly, my grandmother suffered third degree burns and was hospitalized and then moved to a nursing home and was never able to return home again due to multiple reasons. Most significant was her memory problems and inability to recognize her limitations. They called it senility back then. I know now that she had Alzheimer's. I digress here to point out that resistance to having help is not uncommon. I recently was called by a friend, who was at her wits end with her mother, because she did not want anyone helping her at home, except her daughter. Any health aid sent to her home she sent away or when they call to confirm, she tells them she's fine and doesn't need anything. My friend was so frustrated and felt like her mother was the only one who does these things. My friend actually told me that "most people are happy to receive help." This has not been my experience. Letting go of independence is, I believe, one of the most difficult issues of aging along with illness and dementia.

I did not want my aunt to be injured like my grandmother had been. I needed someone else to help me get my aunt to accept assistance. My aunt was in complete denial about the condition of her home, and her own limitations to take care of herself. But first, I needed to become my aunt and uncle's power of attorney.

Attorney, Hospital Visit and Signing of Paperwork

I needed to get a hold of the attorney my uncle had met with a year or so before this crisis. One of the most challenging things about this experience was the rushed timing of everything. I needed to quickly find the attorney to have the paperwork signed and notarized in order for me to take care of my aunt and uncle's affairs, just like what I had to do for my parents. I made phone calls, and drove to the attorney's office. She was at her other office in another town, but agreed to meet me the next day at the hospital. She suggested the meeting be held with me, my aunt and uncle and her assistant in my uncle's hospital room. I had wondered how we would achieve getting everyone together and was so relieved when she offered this option of coming to meet us at the hospital. Fortunately, when I spoke to the attorney before the appointment over the phone she was very reassuring and took time to answer my questions and explain the process and what she hoped to achieve during her visit. A good thing was that she remembered meeting with my uncle and she recalled that my aunt had never signed the paperwork, which included the Living Will, Power of Attorney, and Trust documents. At least we weren't starting from scratch.

On the way to the hospital my aunt was exhausted from getting ready to go as well as from the stress she had been under for quite some time. I dropped my aunt off at the front door of the hospital. She could barely walk, so I found a bench for her to sit down and wait before going back out to park my car. When I came back into the hospital, she insisted that she could walk when I suggested getting a wheelchair. She was not accepting my help and was behaving in an oppositional manner, which I now know was from the dehydration, as well as extreme stress. After her struggling and my holding her up and before I could locate a wheelchair, the elevator came and we rode it up to my uncle's floor. Upon exiting the elevator my aunt collapsed. I was alarmed, yet so relieved that we were in the hospital when it happened.

We were immediately surrounded by nurses, who took her to the emergency room. I told them I needed to check in with my uncle in his room, as we had an appointment with their attorney and gave them the room number and my phone number as well as asked them to keep me posted on her status. On top of her medical concerns I was beginning to understand that my aunt's dementia was more of a factor than I knew until I was actually physically with her, not just talking on the phone. Talking to her on the phone was one thing, being with her from sun up to sun down and watching her world was a real eye opener.

My aunt received an IV with fluids and electrolytes and also medication to stabilize her blood pressure. Fortunately, this helped her enough so that she was able to come to my uncle's room and meet with the attorney and we got all the paper work signed. I had no idea how it would all come together and was so impressed with how the attorney managed the meeting. She was kind, patient and efficient. The fact that my uncle had time to talk with me and the attorney, without my aunt present in the beginning, actually ended up being a good thing. It helped him to relax and by the time my aunt came in, everything was ready for signing. The attorney kindly explained everything to my aunt and she signed the paperwork. She was very shaky and weak but signed. I had learned from my parent's experience that I had to take action when I knew that there was no other choice.

Now that we had signed all of the paperwork necessary for me to help with their affairs, from paying their bills, to becoming their Health Care Surrogate, I was ready to get things done legally, including dealing with their banks and helping to place my aunt in respite care. I could meet with people on her behalf, which made things so much easier. All of this was different because it was not my parents. I had to explain why I was helping them and what my relationship was to them. I was the only one who could step up to help them at this point. Fortunately, they were still "with it" enough to verify what I told them. I was not a money grubbing relative there to take advantage of them, which as we know can and does happen.

The good thing was that deep down, they both knew that I was doing what I was doing out of love for them. Because of our close relationship all along, my swooping in was not strange. I am grateful that we maintained connection even after my moving out of state years before.

CHAPTER TWELVE

SO MUCH TO DO—SO LITTLE TIME

I realized quickly that time had stood still in the condo with things like opening mail, taking or filling prescriptions, cleaning out the refrigerator of dated food, and there were large black Hefty bags of garbage in the living room. The carpet had obviously not been vacuumed for a very long time and the kitchen counters were cluttered and dirty. My aunt actually was using scotch tape to get the cat fur off the carpet. I could not believe what I was seeing when she stooped down to do this. The bed linens and laundry had not been done for a very long time as well. On top of everything else, there was the cat, my aunt and uncle's pride and joy. They loved the cat and I needed to make sure that she was cared for, too!

As with my parents, finding things was not easy. Thankfully, some of the organization that once existed in their lives was still available, which helped me piece things together. Plus, my uncle was able to help me sometimes with what he knew. Not all the time, mind you, but enough to give me some idea of where they banked for example. Unfortunately, banks change names, which can get confusing, especially with safety deposit boxes that need keys. In their case, the keys could not be located and nobody knew where they were. The bank name given to me was wrong, which made for some time consuming and difficult issues along the way. Eventually, I solved the case of the mystery of the lost key and lost bank and managed to get what was needed out of the safety deposit box. Thanks to the Power of Attorney now in place, I could take care of business, which was absolutely critical.

Finding the Right Resources

I not only had lived in the area where my aunt and uncle lived, I had also worked there and was familiar with resources. However, I had been away from this area for twelve years so many things had changed. Despite this, it was comforting to be somewhere I knew, which gave me a head start on things.

One of the first calls that I made was to my aunt's church. I was hoping that someone could go by and check on her but this did not work out for a few reasons. When I called the church I learned that they had offered to visit my aunt to give her communion in the past when she was housebound. Apparently in the beginning, my aunt would meet them at the door, but then reportedly told them not to come inside. With this new information I left a message for the nun my aunt always told me about. She was someone she trusted and often called her "my friend, Sister Betty." This connection proved helpful in that she stayed in touch over time with my aunt via an occasional phone call and visit. Once my aunt was no longer living in her home, she had no problem accepting visitors. I have a feeling my uncle was the one who didn't want people coming inside to see my aunt, because he knew it would show that they were not able to care for their place as they had always done before. I am pretty sure they were also embarrassed.

While lying on my aunt's bed with her amidst a pile of newspapers, tissues and magazines, I asked if we could call her old friend, who used to live upstairs. The address book was in the bed, too. I remember being very worried when I heard she had moved a year or so before, because she and her husband had looked out for my aunt and uncle. One thing they did was to make holiday meals for them and delivered them to their door. Very kind and thoughtful people, whom my aunt adored. What a relief it was when she agreed to call. She dialed her friend who had moved to Florida and told her about my uncle and that I had come to help her. I asked to also speak with her and she willingly handed me the phone to explain more of what was happening and ask if she knew anyone who could help when I wasn't in town. Fortunately, my request for help was met with a name of someone to call. I felt some of the weight lifted off of my shoulders. The name given was a person my aunt knew from her church.

This one phone call led to more supportive help than I ever could have imagined. Just knowing that I could call someone in the area was a relief. Their neighbor called her good friend, and told her the situation. The plan was for me to call the woman, whom I will call MT, so we could set up a time to meet. She was recently retired from teaching and had time to help. Fortunately, the woman knew my aunt and my uncle and was very agreeable to help; a big relief to me. From what I could see, this was not going to be a short-lived situation and I was right.

So now I knew that I would be able to leave for a time to organize my own life. Once again I was traveling back and forth until things settled. This disruption to my life would not have been as bad had I not just moved myself and was not settled. Again, my life felt derailed. I learned a lot with my parents' experience, but it didn't hit all of the same issues in the same way. There was more to learn in this situation.

Calling Adult Protective Services

Never did I think that I would be calling Protective Services to report a concern for a family member, but what I was witnessing was an unsafe environment for my aunt. I wanted help and support for her, because of the condition of the condo and my aunt's health needs and unrealistic view of her situation. My aunt was not technically being abused or neglected. Instead, her living conditions put her at a high risk level for falling, malnutrition, and not being able to take care of her own basic needs. I should add, that awhile back I had suggested to both my aunt and uncle that they consider hiring someone to come into the home to help with cleaning and organizing. They could have benefitted from home health services as well. My aunt refused to even talk about such ideas. This resistance was very familiar, as I met with the same opposition with my parents. It wasn't any easier this time, and in fact maybe even more difficult the second go around.

In my work, I was mandated by law to report any suspected abuse or neglect of a child, so I was familiar with the reporting process, but this was an adult and a relative. I was conflicted about calling, but knew it was my best chance to get the proper help for my aunt, which in my mind was placement in a care facility. The social worker I spoke to on the phone, came to the condo, and fully agreed with my assessment.

Before the person from Protective Services arrived, I prepared my aunt for the upcoming visit and explained that the woman coming to meet with us was a social worker, like me, except helped adults, who could help me to best help her. I was honest and told her that I could not in my right mind leave her alone in the condominium and that my uncle would not be well enough to come home for quite some time. My hope was to take the focus off of me as the person making these decisions by shifting the focus onto the professionals, including her own doctor. I also wanted her to know that I needed help, too, to figure out what to do. She seemed open to this idea, so I was optimistic.

I was extremely lucky that the social worker who came to the house was the perfect person for what we needed. Her name was Carolyn, and she was wonderful--nonthreatening, attentive and very professional. From our telephone conversation, she seemed like a good fit. Before Carolyn arrived, I told her that my aunt was capable of joining our conversation. So before her arrival, I gave my aunt the choice of participating in the discussion or to stay in bed. I knew that my aunt did not want to leave her home, and I knew that her perception about her ability to take care of herself was unrealistic. I hoped that what the social worker said to my aunt would make sense to her and that she'd accept her recommendations.

We ended up having our talk sitting at the dining room table, with my aunt joining us. She was gracious and told Carolyn about her life; who she was and what she had accomplished. I know she wanted to make sure she to let this person know that her life wasn't always like what she was seeing. It was both heartening and disheartening to listen to her stories. I liked seeing her enjoyment around sharing her life, but at the same time I knew that she was telling about what used to be, not what was happening to her now. I grieved both with her and for her. I felt sad and worried, plus completely overwhelmed by realizing what the next steps would be.

While Carolyn was there, she presented a very good option for my aunt called "Respite Care" and gave me the name of the facility, which was nearby my aunt and uncle's home. In this case respite care for my aunt was a placement in an assisted living care facility to make sure she was safe and her medical needs monitored, with three meals a day provided. At this point, this placement was considered to be temporary. I first made arrangements for my own tour of the facility without my aunt. I did not want to put her through a tour before it met with my own approval. I liked what this assisted living facility had to offer so I went ahead and set up an appointment with the Director of the facility to include my aunt for the next day.

Touring the Respite Care Facility

The day of our tour just so happened to be Halloween. When we arrived, all of the staff were dressed in costumes, including the admissions director of the facility/tour guide. She greeted us with a warm, outgoing welcome, complete with a big orange wig and clown painted face. She was inviting and funny all at the same time. This comic relief was just what my aunt and I needed. Because of my aunt's weakness and breathing difficulties, I asked for a wheel chair, which was graciously provided. My aunt didn't want it, but I knew we'd be walking quite a bit and reminded her of what happened while visiting my uncle at the hospital. I used humor to cajole her into accepting the "luxury" of riding in style in a wheelchair. When she was in her small condo, she didn't require the assistance, but in places like the hospital and to tour the assisted living facility she had a very difficult time breathing and walking.

The tour went better than I expected. Part of the tour was the option to have lunch in their dining room. Initially she said, "No!" So, I told her I was hungry and would love to try their food. It worked! While touring and dining she was pleasant and made positive comments about the rooms and the dining room. Much to my surprise, she seemed accepting of the idea of moving in temporarily until my uncle was healed. She even willingly signed papers and gave her insurance cards to the director and said she would move in. I was so relieved. I thought that the facility was perfect for her needs. I already felt strongly that ultimately both my aunt and my uncle needed to move into assisted living, but for now the focus was on short-term respite care for my aunt.

A Change of Mind

In the car on the way home, she was very quiet and seemed like she was mulling over all that she had just heard, seen and experienced. I am sure it was a lot for her to process. It meant a major life change for her, so under-standably difficult to accept. I shared my feelings about the visit and what I thought would benefit her. The lunch had been quite good, the atmosphere very accepting and the rooms seemed to be clean and accommodating for what my aunt and uncle needed in terms of space. And, most importantly, it was pet friendly so she could take her cat with her. I really thought I had, "made the sale." Unfortunately, by the time we got back to her place, she was adamant that she was not going back there and that she would wait for my uncle to come home.

My feelings of relief and hopefulness were quickly dashed. My aunt agreed with me, that the woman who gave us the tour seemed very nice, and that the facility appeared to be very clean and the food was very good. Once she was in the comfort of her own home, she vehemently told me in no uncertain terms that, "I am not going there!" She felt she could handle everything at home by herself. I knew that this was a recipe for disaster. She was afraid that my uncle would be angry with her for leaving their home. She told me that if she left it would, "Kill him."

I realized, even though the place was not a nursing home and offered the perfect place for her to live, "temporarily," her fear was that it meant that her life as she knew it was ending. I knew that she was scared, but found myself feeling frustrated and angry that she wasn't agreeing to the idea of respite care. I sold it as not being permanent, even though I knew deep down that the likelihood of her returning home was low. Deep down she may have realized this as well. Her resistance escalated. She was shouting and so was I. I was at my wits end, exhausted and up against a strong willed woman, who was fighting what I knew in my heart, was the best thing possible for her. It would be easy to feel intimidated by my aunt's complete opposition to my attempts to help her, but I did not waiver.

I was feeling very angry with my aunt at this point and realized I needed to stop arguing, get some distance from her and start thinking of a strategy to deal with her resistance. What she was expressing and feeling was not unusual, but at this moment, because I was so close to her, my response was also filled with emotion, which fueled an already difficult situation.

I went to my own room to give each of us some space and a break. It had suddenly occurred to me that my aunt told me about a year or so before that if she ever went into a nursing home my uncle would leave her. This recollection helped me better understand more about her opposition. Plus, her mother, my grandmother had lived in a nursing home because of her severe dementia. I had to figure out a way to make this happen.

Who, What, Where and How?

It hurt me to see her in such distress in every way possible: failing health, an inability to manage her day-to-day affairs, being apart from her critically injured husband, and living where it was unsafe and unmanageable for her anymore. I called my sister and together we felt the male influence from our aunt's one and only nephew, my brother, might be able to help me convince her to go into respite care. It would be beneficial to have someone support what I was telling her and to be there with me. Thankfully, he was willing and able to help me out.

I realized from working with children and families in my role as a social worker, that it's best not to tell people what to do, but to engage them in the process of problem solving. In this case, I needed my aunt to help me to help her, which I hoped would make her feel less helpless and more involved in getting help. I knew she wanted me to stay with her for as long as it took, but I also knew that this was not realistic or the best choice. I knew that she was very scared of what lay ahead, which was to be expected and understood. I could think all of this through rationally; however, when she would fight me, I cannot say that I was always patient and for this, I still feel guilty. I knew in my heart I was doing the right thing to help her, yet, even knowing what I was doing was helping, not hurting, I second-guessed myself and needed a sounding board, someone like my sister, to check my decisions. It was so difficult to watch how hard it was for my aunt to face the changes ahead for her. It was a very painful process. Achievable, just not easy!

Dealing with Opposition to Moving

With my parents, there was some voiced resistance to moving, but there wasn't a big fight when the time came to actually move into a care facility, mostly because of my dad's stroke. Once he had his stroke, he really didn't have any fight left in him and he went along with the professional's recommendations. My aunt, on the other hand, had some fight left and she wasn't shy about expressing her resistance when the time came to give respite care a try. I found myself getting angry. Regretfully, I remember shouting that she was worse than my dad and her own mother.

Helping someone you're very close to is much more difficult than helping someone who isn't. This situation was emotionally charged for me for sure. She may have been very weak physically, but adrenalin must have been powering her oppositional behavior. I understood her fears and felt for her, but I was admittedly not too patient when the day came that I had to convince her to get in the car to go to the Respite Care facility. I had the added stress of knowing that I had to go back home. This was one of the differences between caring for my parents and caring for my aunt and uncle. I could not see myself staying for weeks like I did for my parents. I felt a sense of urgency to get my aunt into a safe place quickly.

I needed backup so I called my brother and asked him to come down on the day we were scheduled to move my aunt to the respite care assisted living facility and he did. I also called MT to see if she could come assist us, not knowing just how tough it was going to get and she agreed to come, so I accepted her offer. I had no idea how bad it would get. First thing that morning she was cooperative and willing to get ready to go. When the time came to getting into the car, the brakes came on and there was no budging her. She repeatedly said, "I'm not going" refusing to leave her bedroom. I was beyond distraught!

In the meantime, my brother got lost on the way to her place. He must have called me five times for directions. It was a simple route, and I was surprised that he kept passing the turn. I figured that he was nervous about what I had asked him to help me with. I had to sit outside in the cold to get a cell signal to keep talking him in. I felt like my head was going to explode. I called the social worker to let her know how things were going, and she supported my efforts as I waited for my brother to arrive. MT stayed in the house with my aunt. I was exhausted and could not believe all the obstacles to getting my aunt to go to a nice place to stay to keep her safe. My brother finally found the place one hour later. Between all of us, we were able to get my aunt into the car, but easy it was not!

Thank God, once I got my aunt and the cat to the facility, things were calm and she was willing to stay. My aunt's behavior reminded me of some of the kids I had worked with who had separation anxiety and/or school phobia (not wanting to come to school). Big difference being, I was the niece, trying to convince my aunt to leave her home. I know deep down she knew she wasn't ever coming back home.

Going through something like this with my aunt was like "Tough Love." It hurts to do it, but it's far worse to ignore it and hope the problem simply goes away. I understand why some people give up. I know we gave up on my father earlier when we all knew things were bad. Sometimes a crisis is the only driving force to make the changes needed to keep our loved ones safe.

This brings me back to "Hoping for the best and planning for the worst!" It is a good idea, but honestly I know that our good intentions may in fact fail. Getting knowledge ahead of time is important, and being willing to reach out for help from others essential. I believe that if I had not called in Adult Protective Services, I may not have trusted my judgment and might have left feeling defeated. Sure I could have asked someone to check on my aunt, but my guess is she would not have answered the door. I was there, and I decided I would not leave until I made sure my aunt was safe despite her extreme resistance.

Returning Home

Because of commitments back home I had to leave my aunt and uncle. One thing that alleviated some of my worry was that MT agreed to check in with my aunt and uncle and find out what they might need for themselves or their cat. They too knew that they could call her if there was something they really needed in a pinch. This arrangement worked out great and what a relief it was for me. Finding someone who was available and willing and able to be a backup when you're a long distance caregiver is invaluable. The trust factor, as you might imagine is big, so having found someone who was known to my aunt, had the time, and was warm and kind was truly a blessing.

It wasn't so much about them needing things from the store, but more about them not feeling abandoned and helpless. Someone was there to care for their needs in a personal way. My aunt and uncle looked forward to her visits and told me how helpful she was to them. The fact that they welcomed this made things much easier for me. I know that sometimes people push such help away, so their acceptance of MT's help was essential for the arrangement to work. And MT and I spoke before and after her visits and she became a friend and huge support for me as well.

Traveling

The traveling was one of the things I dreaded the most. I suppose if you are a natural born traveler, this part of the "journey" of caregiving might not be so bad. For me it was a challenge. I hated leaving my home and I hated flying and leaving my own plans and life behind. Despite this, I adapted to this new "duty" by accepting some of the more mundane aspects of travel. I found that I began to appreciate some of the smaller pleasures in life when taking the frequent trips to see my family in need. My frame of reference changed during the process of long distance caregiving by challenging my comfort zone and the need for control. I had to learn more patience and become more flexible. This is not to say that I no longer complained at times about the inconveniences of travel attached to crises, but I did learn to make the best of my trips to take some of the sting away.

For example, the 6:00 a.m. breakfast at Chiles Restaurant was something I looked forward to each trip. And, if there wasn't a Chiles there was always Burger King. And, yes, I gained weight during my caregiving years. Food is definitely comforting and with little time to exercise, other than running through airports or up and down hospital hallways, I often found a short-age of energy and time to exercise. I ate comfort food to soothe my soul. I was alone on every trip, so it was easy to drown my sorrows and feelings of loneliness with food. I was not as good at finding healthy ways to assuage my feelings and provide me with outlets that were more constructive. This came over time, not right away. It was a learning process for me. I knew intellectually what was best for me, just couldn't put it into practice con-sistently. I know this is true for others as well. With each experience, came newfound ways to cope, which I will talk about in my brother's story.

Big Changes: Moving My Uncle In With My Aunt

My uncle's stay in the hospital was lengthened due to a bout with what is called, MRSA, which stands for methicillin-resistant staphylococcus aureus. This is similar to a staph infection but resistant to many antibiotics. My most vivid memory about this was that one day when I went to visit him in his hospital room, I was instructed to put on a mask, gloves and a gown before entering his room. It worried me, but the staff assured me that this infection was common and I would be fine. Every patient was tested through a quick swab of the nose.

After he was cleared from infection, he was discharged, not to home, or with my aunt in her assisted living unit, but instead to an inpatient rehabil-itation care facility, where he would stay, I believe, about four weeks. I was quite familiar with what this entailed having gone through this with both of my parents. In my uncle's case, my biggest concern was that his main goal and hope was to go home after he was stabilized,

By the time the transition from the hospital to the rehabilitation center took place I was back in Florida. Thanks to having all of the legal papers in order, I was able to coordinate this by phone with the staff of the hospital, and the staff of my aunt's facility, so that they could support my aunt in knowing and understanding what was happening. My plan before leaving was to get back up to Michigan during the holidays to take care of business and to assist in my uncle's moving in with my aunt.

My uncle's wish to go home after his therapy was not realistic. My aunt was still in the respite care facility and needed to stay there. While he had been in the rehabilitation center my aunt required hospitalization for her own health issues. She was released back to the respite care at around the same time my uncle was ready for discharge. The problem was that my uncle was not ready to go home after he was discharged from inpatient rehabilitation, and my aunt needed to stay in assisted living. I managed to convince my uncle to go live with my aunt in the assisted living facility, as neither one was ready to handle the rigors of living independently after he was discharged from rehabilitation. The condo was not safe to accommodate either one of their physical needs. This was not an easy sell, but I managed, with professional support, to make it happen. And by professional support, I mean the doctor, discharge planner, in this case a social worker, and the therapy staff all concurred that going home was not recommended.

Whenever my attempts to help was not accepted or agreed with, I admit I felt like walking away and letting the "chips fall where they may". I had to dig deep, and take a step back and take a break. Deep down I knew that I was doing the right thing, but when I was met with strong resistance, I doubted myself. As I had learned to do, I checked in with my sister to bounce things off of her to confirm that my plans were sound and in the best interest of my aunt and uncle.

In this case, I first presented to my uncle how well the assisted living facility was supporting my aunt's needs. I told him what they could provide, which couldn't happen at home. My aunt had recently needed hospitalization and was required oversight and assistance. With this, I went on to suggest that he first go live with my aunt in the respite care unit, where he could also benefit from the extra services. I focused my recommendation around my aunt, not him, because I knew that if it was about his health and ability to take care of things, his resistance would increase. I luckily succeeded in convincing him to at least try it until he and my aunt were healthier and stronger again.

Fortunately, the unit my aunt was living in had two very small bedrooms, and a sitting room with two reclining chairs. I ordered two electric medical recliners for them and had them delivered before my uncle was discharged.

Thanks to the Internet, I could do these things from Florida. In addition, since they both loved TV, they had one in each bedroom and one in the sitting room. I brought two from home and one was provided by the facility. In this unit there was also as a handicap-access bathroom. The space was perfect for them. Their home was not handicap access for showering and was not considered to be safe

My aunt was getting used to her new life and I believe it gave her some sense of relief. She didn't love it mind you, but she was able to see the benefits of her easier life. Once my uncle settled in to the small unit with my aunt, he seemed to accept being there more in the beginning. The problem was, when my uncle felt better, the desire for both of them to return home was ignited by my uncle's frustration over his lack of freedom.

Fortunately, Mike, the guy who originally took him to the hospital, would take him to lunch about once a week and even took him to his condo to sit once in awhile. Mike had taken my aunt and uncle's cars to his service station and kept them there. He used my uncle's car to take him to lunch. This went well for quite some time. But, when my uncle became stronger again, he insisted on having his car and keys where he was living in assisted living. This was frightening to me, but I had no way to stop him from driving. I did know that his eyesight was very poor due to cataracts that he never had addressed. I spoke to the director of the facility to see what could be done to keep my uncle from driving. I recall he drove a few times without mishap. However, something did occur one time where he got lost and could not find his way in an area that had always been very familiar to him. He used his cell phone to have Mike come and help him get back to the facility. When I heard what had happened, I asked the director for help. She said the easiest thing to do was to take his car keys and keep them locked up in the facility safe, where his other belongings were kept, such as his wallet.

Shortly thereafter, a new health concern arose that put an end to my uncle's driving by virtue of what happened. While dining out for lunch with Mike, my uncle appeared to be having a stroke. Mike took him to the hospital, where it was determined that he was experiencing "atrial fibrillation" an erratic heart beat that can become extremely fast and lead to a stroke. This meant he needed a prescription to help regulate this heart condition. I presume that my uncle had this for some time, but because he wouldn't go to a doctor, it wasn't detected. My uncle's ignoring of his symptoms and his own health issues is not that uncommon for caregivers. His focus was on keeping my aunt healthy to the detriment of his own health.

Daily Living and Money Management Concerns

In the beginning my aunt tried to manage her bills after moving into respite care. She had her checkbook, and I had established forwarding of their mail, so she received their bills. I wasn't certain if she could manage keeping track of everything, based upon the disarray I found in the condo, but hoped with her daily living needs being tended to, and her medications administered accurately that it was worth a try to help her to retain some independence. Besides, I didn't want another fight and she was adamant that she could handle it, so I figured I would see how it went for a month or two.

After about two months, I discovered that my aunt was forgetting to send payments and her checkbook was making no sense. My uncle had never been the one to pay the bills so having him do this was not an option. What I dreaded most, was having to tell my aunt that we needed to find a better way to make sure that her bills were paid correctly and that things were not lost. During one of my visits, I found stacks of mail that she had never opened, including cards from friends, not just bills. This was a function of her dementia.

To help my aunt accept that she would not be the one to pay the bills anymore, I used the fact that because of her frequent trips to the hospital, keeping track of everything was becoming too difficult. My plan was to set up an account where I was also named on the account to help them stay on top of their finances, using online bill pay and to set up direct deposit of their social security checks. The problem at this point was that the checks they were receiving were not being taken to the bank for deposit unless I was in town to deposit them. This arrangement had an easy fix and that was to sign on for direct deposit by Social Security. After some opposition by my aunt, I was able to convince her of the increased security of such a system. She agreed to give it a try. I presented changes as trials and emphasized that things could be changed back if it didn't work out or if they were able to go back to getting checks in the mail. I knew that this was very unlikely, but I found that it was best not to dash her hopes of gaining back control, knowing this was highly unlikely and that once the system was in place, acceptance would follow.

As with my parents, my power of attorney permitted me to do this, but it was important for me to include my aunt in what was happening, despite her confusion and expected opposition to the plan. I also explained these things to my uncle. He actually was more accepting of my suggestions, knowing that my aunt's abilities to manage everything had been failing. I went to their bank, with their knowledge, and spoke to the bank manager. Because she lived in a small town, they knew her and my uncle well. Also, on the way to the doctors, we had gone through the drive through and my aunt introduced me to the woman at the window. I had all of the proper papers to present and the changes were easily taken care of without too much of a hassle. The logistics were not easy to take care of from afar, however, with modern technology it was manageable; time consuming but doable.

The mechanics of my taking over the control of my aunt and uncle's financial affairs, such as paying the bills, and overseeing their stock portfolios was not the biggest problem I faced. Instead, my aunt's feelings around losing control over her finances was the issue. Through this experience, I learned that in order to minimize conflict with her it was best to focus on the fact that I needed to do this for her and my uncle, because of the situation created by their surrounding health issues at the time. My presentation as to why I needed to step in to help had to stay clear of any focus on her being incapable, or that her memory was too poor to continue. Instead, I talked about her physical health and illnesses, resulting in frequent interruptions in payments and even forgotten or lost payments. I went on to say that situation made it too difficult for her to keep things organized. Her circumstances were the cause of the errors or non-payments, not her incompetence. With my explanations, she moved from adamant opposition, to a place where she accepted this without too much of a problem.

Financial Protection and Oversight

Those who are suddenly ill, elderly or disabled are particularly vulnerable financially. Oversight by someone, be it a family member, or an agency who specializes in such money management is essential. What I had learned from managing my parents' bills surrounding their care, was that there was fairly high risk of inaccurate charging on the part of hospitals, pharmacies (the worst offenders) rehabilitation centers, assisted living, or skilled nursing centers. I often had to make calls to billing departments to have items removed from invoices and bills adjusted. I was shocked by the high number of errors I found. After countless hours on hold and talking to people over the phone, the errors could be corrected, but such changes were time consuming and frustrating. I shudder to think of how many elderly or disabled individuals are wrongly charged and such errors go unnoticed. I felt much better knowing that my aunt and uncle's invoices were reviewed each month by me, which was a protection for them. Living in such facilities is not cheap. It truly is like watching water go down a drain!

On top of the medical bills and residential care invoices, my aunt and uncle's vacated condo was still producing bills for electricity, heat, monthly fees, etc. I vowed to keep them both involved in telling them what I was taking care of and this seemed to appease them. These changes had to be made if I, as a long distance caregiver, was going to be able to protect them from making a major financial error, or from things like theft of checks, and non-payment of bills or delinquent payments.

Once my aunt saw that I could take care of such matters, it actually became a load off of her shoulders and she marveled at the new-age way of doing business via computers and the internet. I told her she would have loved such systems based upon her past career. This would redirect her thoughts to telling me stories of her early computer experiences with the large oil company she worked for. I found that when people feel their independence being "taken away" from them, either because of illness or dementia, the fight is strong to hang on to their control. This, I found, is one of the most challenging parts of caregiving. I felt like I walked around with a knot in my stomach for many years, every time I had to address such issues surrounding my need to takeover financial oversight for those for whom I was caring.

Inaccurate Billing

By the end of 2010 my aunt and uncle's overall care had changed for the worse and the invoices I was receiving were incorrect. When I tried to reach someone to inquire about the obvious overcharges, I was unable to speak to anyone; instead got the run around and was in what I call "transfer-hell." One letter explained the billing department errors as being the result of a changeover in their billing program. As time went on, it became quite apparent that the care was going downhill and the billing was filled with inaccurate charges. The director that I had trusted had left and the new person was pleasant but ineffectual and gave me the runaround, much like the billing office. I felt helpless trying to deal with these problems from afar and resented spending hours on the phone with people on the other end of the line who were dancing around my questions. These issues were inconvenient and annoying, but I had a legal and moral duty to protect my aunt and uncle's health and safety and their money and assets. I felt a very deep sense of commitment about this responsibility.

Another example of where I was able to catch something that was costing my aunt and uncle a great deal of money, was when their electric bills had soared and there was nobody living in the condominium. I actually had a friend who worked for the power company, who was able to expedite an investigation of this incredibly high spike in charges shortly after my aunt and uncle vacated the condo. The investigation discovered that a neighbor upstairs had plugged into their electrical system and had been stealing their power causing the spike in usage and charges. Again, sometimes it's not what you know, it's who you know to get things done. The meter reader had not found this, so an investigator, thanks to my friend, was dispatched. My aunt and uncle were vulnerable for this type of theft. This experience confirmed to me that I was doing the right thing to oversee all of their bills and financial needs.

Juggling and Prioritizing Care Giving Roles

Not too many months later, my aunt told me that there was no longer a nurse on staff. I verified this with a call to the Director of the facility. Unfortunately, I did not have the time to attend to this situation, because of the fact that my brother was diagnosed with cancer in June of that year. I was pulled in two different directions and this meant that I had to prioritize who needed my assistance the most, and at this point, my brother's situation trumped my aunt and uncle's. I will wait to share my brother's story after completing my aunt and uncle's.

I knew that my aunt and uncle's care had changed for the worse. They were both hospitalized more frequently. It was clear that they needed to be moved to a better facility due to a change in management and a decrease in health care. I remember my aunt and uncle telling me that the doctor that came to see them each week, peeked his head in the door, asked how they were, charged them a lot of money and left. This may have not been exactly what was going on, but I believe there was definitely an element of truth in this and of course concern for me.

For now, I will briefly summarize the situation. The fact that my brother needed my help at this juncture in the oversight of my aunt and uncle's care, caused me to be spread thin. And, because of my brother's very serious health issues, I had to back off from my trips to see my aunt and uncle and I had to accept the place where they were living. This made me anxious and worried, but the priority at the time was my brother.

Thankfully, I was able to cope with this shift in attention, without too much guilt, because I knew that my aunt and uncle were comfortable and had become familiar with their routine. Their trips to the hospital had increased and I could find some comfort in knowing that they would be discharged from the hospital, not to their condo, but to assisted living where they were well known by staff and had fairly good care. Not perfect, but adequate. Plus, MT continued to stop in once a week, sometimes twice, bringing them cat food for their cat and any special toiletry they might want/need, or a special snack. My uncle was still able to go to lunch with his buddy, Mike, which gave him some sense of independence.

Nonetheless, there was a six month period, from June 2010 until January 2011 where my focus of oversight shifted primarily to my brother's needs. This meant that my close oversight over my aunt and uncle's lives was cut back and derailed because of another family crisis. Fortunately, because they were in a care facility already, I felt that proper care was in place and I knew that they had a life that had become far safer than what it had been prior to my uncle's fall. On the other hand, I was spread thin, which meant that I didn't notice some things that were of concern with respect to my aunt and uncle, for which I felt badly. In retrospect, things worked out because of the preparation and time spent setting up a new safety net for them. Some things could have been tended to sooner, such as the sale of their condo, had I not been sidelined for what was at the time a more critical family need.

Prioritizing becomes key in these life situations. I was still rattled by my circumstances, but I had learned not to panic as much. I had found a new rhythm in my life. One thing I realize now is that I had an ability to adapt, which is something we all have. What I learned first through my experience with my parents, and then with my aunt and uncle helped me cope a bit better with my next call to action.

Specifically, what became quite apparent was that despite my brother's issues, I had to shift my time and energy back to my aunt and uncle's needs.

They were being cared for. However, they both were becoming weaker, with more signs of dementia as well as serious health concerns resulting in an increase in trips by ambulance to the emergency room. My aunt was being admitted for observation and treatment more often, whereas before, she would be treated in the ER and then sent back to assisted living. My aunt's hospital stays became more frequent and longer. I flew up when I could to see her, but as I mentioned I was spread thin, so had to prioritize.

One convenience and logistical advantage was that when I flew up to help my brother, I could rent a car and drive the two hours to check on my aunt and uncle if the need was vital. This wasn't every time, but each time I divided my time, it took its toll on me physically and emotionally. I felt like a "rat on a wheel" most days and I felt internally torn between needing and wanting to be home and needing and wanting to look out for my family members in need. I had a very difficult time finding joy in my life at the time.

It is difficult at this point to fully separate my brother's story from my aunt's. Given this, without going into my brother's story in depth, I do need to shift here to explain that shortly after my brother's death, my aunt's health plummeted. I know that his passing was devastating for her, as it was for my entire family. I think from the point of learning about his illness, she pushed harder to hang on for my brother and for me. She wanted daily updates and seemed to be able to follow what was happening with him. Despite her poor memory, she always asked about my brother whenever we spoke.

At first, I was very unsure as to whether or not I should share what was happening with my brother. I figured my aunt had certainly lived a long life, which meant she had seen, heard and dealt with all that goes along with it, including, of course, serious illnesses, and losses of loved ones. I am sure that she would have been hurt and angry had I shielded her from the information about my brother. She had a right to know, and for me, it was very important to tell her. After all, she had been my lifelong confidante and mentor in many ways. It also meant that my brother could speak to her over the phone, without pretending that he was fine, when he was not. In retrospect, I have no regrets in telling my aunt about my brother's illness and passing. In this case, honesty was the best policy.

CHAPTER THIRTEEN

THE LAST HOSPITALIZATION: THE FINAL CALL

Shortly after my brother's passing, there came a point when my aunt was hospitalized for approximately two weeks; the longest time yet. Her doctor phoned me, to explain that she did not feel that the hospital was the right place for my aunt any longer based upon her age, prognosis and physical condition. Physically, she was to the point of needing "comfort care," not "curative care." One thing that was different in this case was that my aunt's doctor brought up the option of hospice before I asked for it. The doctor recommended discharge and placement in a long term nursing home/rehabilitation care facility with hospice oversight. She was not responding to medical intervention and was not strong enough to withstand many more trips to the hospital, or any invasive treatment measures. She was now ninety-three and had advanced COPD (Chronic obstructive pulmonary disease).

In my aunt's case, her COPD seemed to be related to exposure to chemicals from her work as a chemist. In the days that she worked, no masks or protection were worn in the lab. She never smoked, but did live with smokers growing up. And since she lived at home until her early forties, she was exposed to second-hand smoke much of her life. Chemical exposure was considered to be the cause of her breathing issues and resulting heart issues as well as her advanced age.

My aunt was discharged to a long-term skilled nursing center/rehabilitation facility, per the doctors' and hospital discharge staff's recommendation. At the same time, my uncle also needed far more care than what was being provided; fortunately, he was able to move in to the facility with my aunt. With some kind-worded urging, I was able to convince my uncle that it was best for him to go where she was and this was permitted by the facility. They were able to share a room in the beginning. My uncle was experiencing many health concerns and had also been in and out of the hospital, so things came together better than expected. Seems odd to be happy about this kind of thing coming together, but what I was relieved about was that they could be in the same place, in the same room and have their medical needs better met.

Of course, this meant me moving them. I recall the feeling of remorse and resistance to flying up to Michigan to move everything out of their living unit. Although it wasn't large, the task was filled with sadness. My next job was to deal with selling their condominium, which was yet another loss; another ending.

Preparing to Sell the Condo

Between my uncle's hope to move back home, and my not having the time to devote to doing what needed to be done to put the place on the market, taking care of this task was long overdue. It was in many ways reminiscent of my parents move, in that, they too had never thrown anything away. On top of personal items accumulated they had a basement filled with things accumulated from a business closed years beforehand. I knew I was in for another overwhelmingly difficult move. Thankfully, I found people to help me again. I was getting much better at asking for help. I will spare most of the details, but one thing that was different than what we did for my parents, was that I took out what was salvageable, or sentimentally charged and placed these items in storage in the spring before the condo was put on the market. My husband had urged me a number of times to do this, but I was so overwhelmed I kept putting it off. I didn't want to admit that I was facing another loss and I was not ready to accept it emotionally. I knew it was inevitable at an intellectual level, but I didn't have the heart to do it. My other obstacle was that I was preoccupied with my brother's needs.

I had just recently lost my brother and was tying up loose ends there and now was faced with what seemed like a monumental task. I was emotionally and physically drained and overwhelmed. My life once again was waylaid, and I felt robbed of my ability to do some of the things I wanted to do. Despite the help I was receiving from others, it still meant countless phone calls and time spent coordinating and figuring out schedules and what to donate, etc. My nephew came through once again, this time with his wife. They came to help me sort through things and take special items that they wanted.

I am much better at throwing things away after moving so many people who never (maybe a slight exaggeration) threw anything out. They were not at the hoarding level, but pretty close to it. Making decisions and cleaning up years of saving and non-disposal was challenging for me. Prior to my friend's nephew coming to the rescue to do final cleanup disposal and placement of items into a storage unit, my nephew weeded through the salvageable items and we donated what was useful, and the rest was taken care of by my friend's nephew.

My learning to talk to people about my situation and/or predicaments, always led to solutions. It is worth the risk to share with others what you are struggling with or what you need and it's worth accepting the help they may offer. Granted, I found out that some people did not want to get involved for reasons that I may never know or understand. What I know now is that dwelling on why some help and some people don't is generally based upon their own issues, and I learned not to take it personally. I can't say I always succeed at this, but that's okay. I know that some families are good at planning ahead and actually are proactive about giving things away and/or disposing of things before they are unable to participate in this part of life. If nothing else, my experiences with my family members, has taught me that if there is any way to plan ahead do it.

Long Term Hospice Support/Care

As the health care surrogate, I was the person who filled out the paperwork and was interviewed so my aunt could be accepted as a hospice patient. My experience with my aunt's hospice care company was really great. What made them special was their system was well organized, the staff compassionate and well trained and their communication with family exceptional. Her care in the skilled nursing center, along with hospice support made for a care experience that provided comfort, volunteer visitors and appropriate medical care at this point in her life. She received hospice care for approximately one year and was reevaluated every three months as was standard. In some cases, as in the case of my uncle, he was placed under hospice care and upon a review of progress he actually "graduated" from hospice care and was placed back under skilled nursing care in the long-term care facility where they were living.

As with both of my parents, hospice was the choice seen as best for my aunt upon hospital discharge. This time I knew more of what to expect. What I learned is that no two hospices are alike and this was no exception. I will share a negative experience I had and what I learned, with a hospice experience I had with my uncle as I relate his story in the next chapter. However, for my aunt hospice care was exceptional. After about a year, she was assessed periodically to determine whether or not she continued to qualify for hospice care. Fortunately, even though she had beaten the odds and survived far longer than was expected, they agreed to keep her as a patient, knowing that the benefits to her far outweighed the discharge guidelines.

The Final Call/My "Driving" Desire to Be There

It was Labor Day, 2012, when I called my aunt's skilled nursing center to check to see how she was doing. It was then that I learned that she had taken a turn for the worse and it sounded like death was imminent. The day before I couldn't reach anyone to talk to; a Sunday, the worst day to find someone to get information. I knew right then that I must get on the road as soon as possible to see my aunt and be there for my uncle when she passed. I made it, but not quite in time. She had passed forty minutes prior to my arrival. I had called a bit before then to let the nurse know that I was close and she put the phone to my aunt's ear and I told her that I would be there for my uncle. I know that this would be what she wanted.

When I finally arrived, it was about 7:30 pm. I ran into the nursing home. Traffic had delayed me, not to mention that I had to get across a bridge that had been shut down most of the day for a Labor Day walk. I wanted to be there for my uncle and once I was with him, I knew that my push to get there was worth it.

My aunt had passed and was left uncovered. She was still in the bed and my uncle started to cry when he saw me and said, "She's gone, she's gone," over and over again. The facility nurse and the aide on duty on this holiday, were not people I knew. Sadly, the hospice nurse who had supported my aunt since the beginning was too ill herself to be there. She had become quite close to my aunt, as it seemed most who cared for her did. She was very well liked, much like my mother. The shock when someone we love has died is so profound. Until experienced, I honestly don't believe that anyone can predict their reactions. What I do know is for me it took my breath away each time.

I like to think that my aunt spared me from watching her die, much as my father did. In my mom's case I wanted to be there. For my aunt, I knew my uncle would prefer his privacy with her, so it worked out for the best. I was there to console him and share in our grief, which was comforting for both him and myself.

My Aunt's Wedding Ring

As with any death, someone has to take care of the details. This was now my third time doing so. We had everything prepared and taken care of ahead of time, so this wasn't like a sudden loss. One unsettling moment, was when at some point, it was discovered that my aunt's wedding band was missing. I believe my uncle noticed this. We never found it and the staff looked through the linens and everywhere in the room. My guess is that it was stolen from her. I never took action on this, because to me it wasn't worth the hassle. It was sad to lose it, but losing my aunt was far more important than a piece of jewelry. My uncle felt the same. We reported it but never heard anything more about it, which was okay with us. Sometimes we need to let things go.

From this point forward, I felt a strong need to stay in touch with my uncle. I loved him and I felt so badly that he was now alone. He had no other family and to be without my aunt was a very difficult absence. I worried about him every day. I knew that I must carry on as his long distance caregiver, not out of obligation, but from a place of love, respect and empathy.

The Arrangements: My Uncle's Legacy

In making arrangements for my aunt's cremation at a local funeral home, I had an uplifting experience with the director of the home. It was a longstanding family owned business, and the man I met with was the son of the original owner, or perhaps grandson, I am not positive. Anyway, I learned what my aunt and uncle meant to some people from this meeting. I had remembered the people who owned the home, had been members where my uncle was a golf pro many years before. I had worked for them while still in college and recalled the son had been a star golfer. Turns out, the director was that young man, who I remembered by name and by my uncle talking about his talents and abilities as a golfer.

The meeting began as one might expect with words of condolences and my feeling deeply sad about the loss of my aunt. When the director looked at the name, the conversation turned to what my aunt and uncle had meant to him and what a positive influence my uncle had been for him. He told me how, because of my uncle's gifted teaching, he was accepted by multiple schools on a golf scholarship, yet chose one out west. His memories of my aunt and uncle were very positive and he spoke from the heart.

I was able to go back to the nursing home and tell my uncle all that was said and what a difference he must have made in so many young people's lives. I know he made a difference in mine. And, of course, we talked about my aunt and how she also was a big part of their "team," all through their years together. I think the one phrase that stuck with me most was when the man said to me, "I cut my golf teeth on your uncle's teaching. He taught me better than anyone else did or has since." This turned into a bittersweet meeting for me. My father's sister had just died; the last relative that we knew from my father's family

The positive memories that this person had of my aunt and uncle helped ease my pain. This connection also paved the way to another benefit. We wanted to wait to bury my aunt's cremains until my uncle passed. The funeral director offered to keep her urn until then. He told me this was a courtesy that they never provided, but in this case he would make an exception. You see, my aunt never told me what their specific wishes were for burial. I actually had gotten up the nerve to ask her at one point and her answer was evasive. I decided to take the offer and leave the cremains there until they could be buried together. Where this would be was still undetermined. Because I spoke openly to the funeral home director about our dilemma, a solution was offered, which my sister agreed to as well. Knowing this was a relief to me.

The nursing home chaplain, who visited my aunt weekly, offered to hold a small memorial in my uncle's room, which turned out to be very special and important to myself and my uncle as well as a few staff members whom she had touched. My uncle, who never had any church affiliation, was open to this offer. He knew it's what my aunt would have wanted. She was very devout, yet never foisted her beliefs onto her husband. In the end, I know that this service symbolized her life of faith. My uncle's love for my aunt rose above their belief differences. I respected this and was touched by how my uncle, laying in his bed in the nursing home, participated in prayer and remembrance of a long life lived well. Where they both would be buried together would be decided when the time came.

CHAPTER FOURTEEN

MY UNCLE'S STORY

My uncle was now my fifth caregiving experience from afar and, although we were very close, he was not my "blood relative." To me, this was not an issue, but I found that sometimes others people's perception of my investment in helping him was one of curiosity. This was not the first time I experienced some judgment on the part of others about why I would do what I was doing. I learned early on that I really did not need to explain the "whys" to others. For me, he was a very important person in my life and married to an aunt, who was like a mother to me. This pretty much summed it up, and really nothing else mattered. What I did find was that the nursing home staff and doctors very much appreciated that someone was there for their patient. They would comment about how many have nobody in their lives who ever visited or called them.

After my aunt's passing I stayed in touch via telephone with my uncle as well as the staff who cared for him. I made a point to connect frequently with nurses and even the receptionist at the front desk. She had her finger on the pulse of all happenings on the floor. She wasn't a nurse but knew what was what on any given day. The staff was sensitive to his needs and had grown to know him well. One male nurse in particular was especially good at letting me know if my uncle needed anything. From my prior experiences, weekends never were as good in terms of care and attention. As with my aunt, I phoned my uncle each day, which he appreciated and counted on. His health was very fragile and his dementia was getting worse. Another concern was that the staff who cared for him, like with my mother, predicted he would most likely die shortly after the loss of my aunt. Like my mother, this proved to be wrong.

One Year Later

After a year by himself in the nursing home, with only one or two visits from anyone within a year's time, my husband and I talked about the importance of going to see him on our way back to Florida. During our short visit, we had taken him in his wheel chair for a walk, which he enjoyed. It seemed to really lift his spirits. When we got in the car, my husband said to me, "We cannot leave him here to die alone." I agreed. We decided to look into finding a facility to meet his needs near our home. We had a place in mind that was a mile from us, which we had actually looked into when my aunt and uncle first needed twenty-four hour care.

The logistics of the move were understandably challenging and took a great deal of my time and energy. We were able to move my uncle into the facility by the end of October, of 2013. It had been just over a year since my aunt had died. And, like my aunt, he vacillated back and forth between wanting to move and telling me he definitely didn't want to move. I, of course, consulted with my uncle's doctor, and anyone who cared for my uncle in the facility and it was unanimous that everyone felt that his being near us was an excellent idea. His health was declining, his dementia worsening and, because he was lonely, the decision was easy to make.

Above and Beyond the Call of Duty

The day I went to pick up my uncle from Michigan for the move to Florida, there was plenty of stress around logistics and worry about how he would do on the long trip. He had not done much of anything for a long time. Fortunately, I had the help of my nephew and the support of the facility staff saying goodbye. The supervisor of the floor had recently been transferred to another section of the facility, but because he loved my uncle so much, he offered to ride with him in the van. In addition, my favorite receptionist accompanied my uncle to the airport as I followed in my rental car. Without their support, I know my uncle would not have gotten into the van. They knew this too, and came along to help ease his anxiety and fear. They went above and beyond the call of duty. The receptionist cried and hugged me hard and told me that I was doing the right thing. The supervisor, told my uncle that he was, "Superman" and that he could handle anything.

A Great Beginning!

As we had planned, my nephew agreed to help me fly my uncle down to Florida. He met me at the airport as scheduled and our rendezvous worked out well. I returned my rental car that I had picked up the day before when I flew in, and then went to find my nephew, who was waiting at the curb when I walked up. I had left slightly before the van left the nursing home and reassured my uncle that I would meet him at the airport. Luckily it all worked like clockwork. When my uncle saw me, I heard him scream out my name from the inside of the van.

The experience of getting through the airport was physically stressful, but we managed. He seemed to enjoy the stimulation of the journey itself and seeing the modern airports and jets. He always drove to Florida and told me he hadn't flown for many years.

As with anything, things don't always go as planned no matter how thoroughly we have prepared. Our first big problem was that the wheel chair transport was too small for my uncle. He was 6'2"; information that I provided ahead of time, but the wheel chair provided was far too small, but they didn't have one to fit him at the time. Our issue with the "wheel-chair" transport onto the plane actually delayed us, hence the flight. As you might imagine, people were staring at us, not with compassion, but with a look of impatience. Somehow, we were able to transfer him into his seat, which was at the bulkhead (seating reserved for disabled flyers). The airline couldn't guarantee this seat, but since he was unable to walk unattended, he qualified. A sense of relief came over me when I finally got my uncle into his seat. Departing the plane went more smoothly. This time they had the proper wheel chair to fit down the jet aisle. Despite all of this, the flight went fairly smoothly and my uncle enjoyed it. He slept much of the way, but when he would wake up we'd talk about the view he saw out the window and I answered his questions about when we would arrive.

My uncle was quiet and very agreeable the entire trip. He never became agitated. He wore adult diapers, and when he needed to use the public restroom my nephew was able to assist him. We were nervous about this, but it all worked out okay. My husband greeted us at the facility where I had arranged for him to move to in Florida, and the Director of Admissions gave him a big hug as soon as he got out of the van that picked us up, which was provided by the facility that he was moving into. The marketing director also greeted with a hearty welcoming hug. All seemed positive at this point. We had bought him some furniture for his room with his credit card and had his TV activated. He seemed okay with the set up and the idea of living near us. I was feeling quite confident that this was the right decision at the right time for my uncle.

Unexpected Behavior

There were some immediate concerns regarding the room and the bed. The TV, although activated and connected to Comcast, was not working. And, my uncle's bed was far too short for his needs. To get the right sized bed did not happen until Monday, and this was Saturday. This seemed annoying, but something that could be solved and was already being addressed.

Choosing this facility and level of care had been done carefully, with much research. My uncle's move from a skilled nursing center to assisted living with "Extended Congregate Care," seemed like a good choice as it provided the insulin injections that he required for Diabetes, something hard to find in Michigan. We hoped this place would offer more stimulation. What we found out rather quickly, was that my uncle needed much more supervision than anticipated. We didn't know just how badly my uncle's adjustment would be on his first night alone. And, we didn't know about some of my uncle's behavioral issues. The paperwork completed by the prior nursing home in Michigan did not mention anything about disruptive behaviors.

Agitation, Confusion, Dashed Hopes

My hopes of a smooth adjustment ended quickly when I phoned the facility the next morning, to ask how my uncle was doing. I was told that he yelled and screamed all night long. His room although nice, private and quiet, was the furthest room from the nurses' station, at the very end of the hall. My first thought was to offer to hire an aide to sit with him the next night. I planned to stay until around 10:00 p.m. and then I would use an outside agency person. This was quite expensive but important and worth it until we could determine if it helped him feel more secure, and to see if this type of living arrangement fit his current needs. I prayed that his behavior was based upon adjustment and that when he became more familiar with the staff and his surroundings that he would stop yelling.

What we didn't know, until I called the prior nursing home to ask about whether or not he had done this with them, was that this behavior was frequent while under their care. He even shouted the same exact words in the previous home, "Help me, help me," over and over. This was very upsetting.

As it turned out, the transfer package of information regarding my uncle's needs had left out all behavioral concerns. I suppose this helped me get him in to the facility, but the downside was he was in a new place that he was unable to handle. I was open to working with the facility nurses and supervisors and asked for suggestions as to what we could do to help him to adjust to his new surroundings. I knew we couldn't pay for a full-time aide as well as the assisted living fee for long. On top of the monetary concerns, I felt badly for my uncle and was desperate to figure out a way to solve this problem.

Misinformation—More Problems

Backing up a bit to my initial screening interview with the Marketing Director, I was assured that any prescription that my uncle had could be delivered upon his admittance to the facility. I was unable to bring his pain medication and anything narcotic, except for, I believe two pills to last him twenty- four hours. We were also given a supply of medication that would last less than a week's time.

Come to find out, I was told that the next delivery was on the following Wednesday. This poorly handled medication transfer led to a beginning that created problems for my uncle, the family (me), the nurses, aides and the other residents who had to listen to my uncle's screaming. He was in pain, and I believed was going through withdrawal. I was told that there was nothing that they could do until the resident doctor came the following Wednesday. This was a predicament that left me with very few options. In retrospect, I could have contacted an Ombudsman, but didn't want to start out this way with the facility. I tried other avenues to see if there was another way to get what my uncle needed.

Unfortunately, it was now the weekend and the supervisory staff was off for the weekend. The nurse on the floor called for assistance and was becoming just as frustrated. We formed an alliance and she became a big support for me and tried her very best to find a solution. I appreciated her compassion, but also saw how exasperated she was as well. This was a great example of poor communication and system breakdown. My hope is that by reading this you may be able to avoid this type of situation. Check and verify medication transfer across state lines and also consider not moving someone on a weekend if at all possible. We didn't have a choice in this situation. Timing is everything.

Adjusting To Dementia

Adjustment for dementia patients, when changes in routine occur, is typically a challenge. We knew it was a risk to take him out of the environment he had become accustomed to, but based on the reports of the Michigan facility we were assured that it was still worth moving him close to family. With his dementia he never had a problem recognizing us. His confusion was based upon what we found out later was atrophy of the brain, vascular issues from diabetes and heart problems from a fibrillation (irregular heart beat). As I prepared to write about my uncle's behavior, I researched what the cause of such behavior might be. I don't recall if I did this when it was happening, except to find out information about the drug Haldol (Haloperidol) that the doctor prescribed, a very old anti-psychotic drug. I knew about the drug from my social work training and background.

In the case of my uncle, I understood that the facility wanted the screaming to stop quickly, and I cannot say that I blame them. It can be upsetting to other patients, residents and staff. My search for information indicated that the behavior is somewhat of a mystery and that medications fall short of eliminating the shouting and screaming behavior in the elderly population. There seems to remain a lack of agreement about what works and what doesn't and why. Of course the patient themselves are obviously in distress, even if they are unable to identify what is wrong. For example, oftentimes when I walked in to see my uncle, I could hear him as soon as I got to his hallway. When I would get to the room, I would ask him, what do you need, or what do you want, what is wrong, or what can I get for you?

He oftentimes would look at me and say, "I don't know. I have no idea!" It seemed to be habitual in nature.

What I read points to the fact that such screaming and/or wailing can represent feelings of physical pain, mental pain and depression, loneliness and/or deep anxiety. Also, that the creative, nonpharmacological approaches often take more time for staff than what may be realistic in a nursing home or memory unit. The articles I read confirmed for me that my uncle's yelling out was a symptom of his loneliness, grief, fear and anger. Whenever he could talk to me about what he was feeling, he expressed deep depression as he said to me, "I want to die. I do not want to be here anymore." He was suffering deeply. And honestly, nothing I or anyone else did alleviated his pain. As long as I was in his room, he was okay. Being around such behavior is exhausting and very sad. The staff and I were affected as well as other residents and their family members.

Moving to the Memory Unit

By the third morning, I was met at the door by the Marketing Director. She walked with me and said, "We have a problem. Your uncle is still crying out all night long and he fell while trying to get to the bathroom in the early morning after the private aide left." She told me that my uncle was considered to be at high risk and not appropriate for the assisted living setting. I understood her point but at an emotional level I did not want to accept what she was saying. Despite this feeling, when she suggested that we move my uncle to the memory unit until he could adjust to his new surroundings, I agreed. I wasn't happy about it, but I understood where she was coming from.

I knew about the memory unit, because when I first visited the facility to decide whether or not it would be a good fit for my uncle, I was taken into the Memory Unit as part of the general tour. It was certainly something to consider and important for me to see. My initial introduction to the unit began by entering through locked doors. I met the staff and saw some of the residents in the unit and immediately felt that it was more than what my uncle needed. My uncle's dementia was indeed an issue, but he seemed more alert, aware and socially engaged than the residents I saw that day. The staff-to-patient ratio was much higher than the congregate care assisted living side of the facility, but everything else I saw indicated that it was too restrictive for his needs.

Most of the residents appeared to be out of it or non-communicative. There was one patient wandering around with a baby doll in her arms, saying inappropriate things. Others were sitting at a table staring into space or an aide was spoon feeding them. Now, the director was telling me that this is the place he needed. I asked if this move could be considered a trial or temporary while he settled into his surroundings, to which she agreed.

Right away, I was concerned by the fact that again he was at the end of the hallway. I hoped that this being a much smaller unit, with ten rooms, designed in a "T" configuration so that staff was always within earshot and had less distance to get to a patient quickly. We found out with his yelling for help, they could hear him from anywhere. He never had mastered the use of the call button, which to me is one of the ironic pitfalls of dementia care facilities that still use this method for calling for help. Nonetheless, I knew that he needed to be somewhere that was more equipped to manage his confusion and behaviors. And, honestly, I was afraid that the other alternative was that he would be asked to leave.

Another difficulty for me in accepting the memory unit was reports by others that my uncle appeared to be free of any problems or social issues at times. He was most often conversant and seemed oriented. Right after my uncle was moved to the memory unit, the daughter of another resident and her husband approached me. They wondered why my uncle was there. She told me her mother, who had been there a year was completely out of it, yet my uncle seemed, "normal" and she and her husband had a great conversation with him.

I explained that he was not always confused, but that there were times that he screamed for help non-stop and was verbally combative with staff. His behavior had been upsetting to the residents and he was at high risk of hurting himself from falling. I added that things didn't work out on the assisted living side and that we are trying to see if the smaller setting would help him to adjust to his new "home" and surroundings. Not too long after this, I saw the couple again and they told me that they could not believe that my uncle was the same person they had seen two weeks prior. This time he was screaming for help and could not be consoled. Conversations like these made me question my decision and made me uncomfortable.

My uncle's behavior in the memory unit did not improve. The staff became frustrated. Once again, I felt like I was being blamed for my uncle's behavior and his constant yelling. When I saw the disturbed looks on the faces of those caring for my uncle as they told me what my uncle had done that day or night before, I felt guilty, even though I knew that his behaviors were not the result of something I was or was not doing. I felt pressure to fix the problem somehow. I logically knew that I couldn't solve it without collaboration with those who cared for him. I understood their frustration and knew that even for me, listening to him for even a short period of time was agitating and extremely frustrating. The plan by the nurse supervisor at this point was for the resident doctor to see my uncle to "treat" his behaviors. I agreed that this was a good idea, but things did not go the way I had hoped.

My Uncle's First Doctor Visit

I wanted to make sure that I was there the day my uncle was examined by the doctor and I was told to be at the facility around 1:00 p.m. on a Wednesday. I visited with my uncle in his room while we waited for the doctor to arrive. The doctor came in and engaged my uncle in conversation. He shouted loudly, which I thought was because all of his patients were elderly and hard of hearing. His first words were, "So you're a veteran?" I realized that he was trying to establish rapport, but then he proceeded to talk about himself and his family history. He bragged about his roots in the area. Interesting to a point. What I didn't appreciate was that he stood at the foot of the bed and never examined my uncle. The doctor never listened to his heart, took his pulse or touched him in any way. My uncle perked up and was friendly and answered his questions. However, mostly it was a monologue. The doctor did not ask me anything, nor did he acknowledge my presence.

One thing that the doctor was obsessed with was a growth on his face, just below his eye. This had been there for years. At the hospital and other facilities he had been, the doctors felt that it was much too risky to remove it and opted to leave it alone. This resident doctor told him he had cancer and that it must be taken care of and that he would arrange an appointment with a dermatologist. He told him where his office was located and that it was something that must be looked at. That was the last he said and out the door he went. I was not impressed and was very annoyed.

From this point forward, my uncle was obsessed and preoccupied and worried by what the doctor had said. He told everyone that he had cancer and that it could travel into his eye and cause blindness. I was so angry after this visit that I went to the Nurse Supervisor to meet with her directly. I wondered if there was another option for a physician and was told that there were no other doctors, unless he were to leave the building to see someone else in the area. The staff didn't discourage my uncle going elsewhere to see another doctor. However, they explained that they used him as their "resident physician," which meant that he was easy to reach when an emergency arose or they needed a medication prescribed or filled quickly.

It was early in my uncle's stay, so I decided to give it time and would try to meet with him privately after he'd had more time to adjust to his new surroundings. I did tell the nurse supervisor that I was told in Michigan not to bother with removal of the growth under his eye due to location and his advanced age. She agreed. I also told her that I wanted some time with the doctor without my uncle present and she suggested again that I come and wait on a Wednesday afternoon to see if I could catch him. No appointment could be made. The doctor's goal it seemed was to see patients in the facility quickly and not have to deal with the family. I was determined to stay involved despite the obstacles; it seemed vital to his receiving proper care.

Prescribed Medication Causes Medical Complications

Within about a week, despite added time for adjustment, my uncle continued to scream and yell. The next Wednesday he would be back and as suggested I went to try to catch him in his "office," which was basically a closet with a desk and one chair. I poked my head in to speak with him as soon as he was available and discovered that my input, questions and concerns were not welcomed or valued at all.

The doctor never looked at me and proceeded to tell me that the nurses wanted him to "do something" to help. He told me that he would be prescribing Haldol to decrease my uncle's behavioral issues, i.e. agitation and repetitive calling out for help. He added that he was at times also combative with aides. I questioned the doctor, because I knew that Haldol was an older antipsychotic drug used primarily for schizophrenia. I had already begun researching the use of this drug for the elderly and found that its use was contraindicated for the elderly population. When I mentioned this to him, he avoided eye contact and said, "It's the best and it would make the nurses happy." I again expressed concern and he said that he could perhaps try a different medication first. I followed up with the nurse supervisor and found out that Haldol had been prescribed anyway.

After a few days, his yelling and screaming was reduced but his physical health was jeopardized and his personality was gone. And, in between doses, he still yelled and screamed. I began asking if the nurses noticed a big change in my uncle's personality? What I found out was that they were happy with his quiet behavior and the fact that he slept all day. Then another new symptom appeared after Haldol was prescribed. His lower legs and feet had swelling (edema) along with weeping fluid from his pores. I reported my concerns to the nurse supervisor and she suggested that the doctor see him again that Wednesday.

Long story short, the doctor completely ignored my observations and my questions as to whether or not the medications he was on, along with the newly prescribed antipsychotic could be at the root of his sudden health decline. He never touched his legs or checked his pulse or heart. He sat on the windowsill during this "exam" and denied any connection to what I saw and possible medication interactions. And, he never acknowledged this new symptom of fluid retention, slurred speech and inability to feed himself.

I made sure that it was now on record that I was concerned by what I saw and the rapid decline in my uncle's alertness and health. I asked my husband to come see my uncle with me to see if my perceptions were accurate. He confirmed my fears and then some. He was angered and saddened by what he saw and told me we must do something. He said, "Your uncle is completely out of it." What is he on? What he had seen was my uncle slumped over at a dining table with a nurse trying to spoon feed him.

I did more research on the medications that my uncle was taking and found that, "It may increase the risk of death when used to treat mental problems caused by dementia in elderly patients." There was also a strong contraindication to take when a patient has a heart condition. I found this warning on the Internet attached to the side effects of the drug itself. And, it was the first side effect listed.

I then recalled the comment the doctor had made about making the nurses happy, and went back to the nursing supervisor with two articles in hand to support my concerns. At this point, I became extremely worried about the politics of what I was up against. I left my meeting with her and realized that although she agreed with my concerns and felt they were valid, she seemed reticent to intercede. I considered filing a formal complaint, but first thought I should talk to another nurse who cared for my uncle to gather some more information.

Calling the Night Nurse

That night, I decided to contact the night shift nurse to find out if she was seeing any changes in my uncle's behavior. I reached her at midnight and shared with her that I was very worried about my uncle's decline in health. The night nurse took a risk and told me that she was worried, too. She shared with me that she would sit with my uncle during the night, and there were quite a few times that he told her that he wanted to kill himself. She shared that she had time to sit with my uncle to talk to him in the middle of the night when he was restless, which helped him feel more secure. The day nurses had less time for this type of personal care and support for the patients.

Hearing how understanding, caring, and dedicated she was gave me an opening to tell her my worries and concerns about my uncle's medical care. She also was the first one to agree that she noticed a change in his affect, demeanor and physical health. She was just as concerned as myself. I knew I had to do something as soon as possible and I had an idea who might be able to help me.

My Doctor Friend Offers Help

My neighbor and friend, who lived across the street from me, just so happened to be a physician, who was a geriatric specialist and he also covered a psychiatric unit in the city. I decided to reach out to him to see if my concerns were warranted with respect to my issues with the resident doctor and the changes in my uncle's behavior and medical status. He thankfully agreed to help and suggested I bring him the list of my uncle's prescribed medications. I also added my uncle's medical profile.

As he reviewed the records, he expressed distress and concern and told me that most of the medications should be removed. They were obviously causing detrimental interactions and side effects and he verified what I had found in my research, that in fact, some should never be administered to elderly patients. He was a proponent of fewer medications for the elderly as they approached end of life. He was the first to tell me that he probably did not have much more time to live based upon his blood work, kidney function and heart issues. In addition, he knew of the doctor treating my uncle and validated my perceptions. The doctor knew the owners of the facility where my uncle lived very well. This was one more situation where it was who I knew that helped me get honest answers and help. This, of course, is not always possible. Nonetheless, it is very beneficial to ask questions when we doubt the care of someone we are helping. And, if possible, obtain a second opinion.

In this case, my doctor neighbor friend suggested he himself provide a "second opinion" by going to see my uncle the next day in the facility. He also offered to be his physician. Unfortunately, my friend never got to see my uncle the next day because that very night, the same nurse, whom I had just talked to a night or two before, called me around midnight to inform me that she had called 911 and my uncle was taken to the hospital.

Contacting the Emergency Room/Advocating for Change in Doctor

I called the emergency room right away to let them know that I was the contact person and to check on my uncle's status. My contact information was on the paperwork, which the facility automatically sends with any patient going to the hospital, but I have found that my calling myself resulted in quicker communication and gave me the opportunity to share what I knew. My experience has been that hospital emergency staff appreciate the information. I was told that my uncle would be undergoing quite a few tests through the night and it was best I wait till morning to come see him. Plus, they connected me with my uncle so that I could tell him that I would be there in the morning. At this point he was "stable."

I saw this emergency room visit as an opportunity to get a second opinion regarding his health and medication needs. I told the ER staff member that I was very concerned about the medications my uncle had been prescribed and that I was unhappy with the facility "resident physician" and requested that someone else could be assigned to his case while he was in the hospital. The person at the other end of the line tried to dissuade me from not using the facility/resident physician. I asked again what choice I had if I did not want the facility doctor to follow my uncle in the hospital and emphatically explained that I felt that his care had jeopardized my uncle's health. I increased my adamancy and stated that I refused to have him be his doctor while in the hospital and asked who else I could speak to in order to make this happen. At this point, her resistance shifted to offering me the option of using their "hospitalist" to oversee and manage his care while he was an inpatient. I was unfamiliar with the term hospitalist so I asked what a hospitalist was, and she gave me a vague definition. Still wanting to know,

I looked it up on the Internet to find out what a hospitalist was and did. Basically a hospitalist is focused solely on hospital care for the acutely ill.

This was not an easy request and judging by the resistance on the part of this staff member what I asked was something not often done. The problem was rooted in the fact that the facility doctor had privileges with this local hospital, therefore it was a very politically sensitive request on my part not to use him. I realized that what I asked was unusual but did not let the intimidation of the staff person stop me from sticking to my request. Fortunately, my request for a change in doctor turned out to be the best thing I could have done for my uncle for more reasons than one.

Visiting my Uncle/Meeting the Hospitalist

The next morning I visited my uncle in his hospital room after checking in at the nursing station. I explained that if possible I would like to speak to the hospitalist and they agreed to page him. They directed me to my uncle's room. When I entered his room, I saw that he was hooked up to IV's and monitors and looked very frail, yet despite this, he actually looked better than he had. He was dozing but woke up and was glad to see me when I said his name. He seemed more alert than he had the day before at the facility, where he could not even feed himself.

Within minutes of my arriving to the room, the "hospitalist" came and told me their preliminary findings and what the current recommendations were for my uncle's care. At this point, the hospitalist was waiting to speak to the cardiologist about the cardiac test results. Most significant was that he had already ordered a discontinuation of many of the medications that had been prescribed by the resident physician from the facility. And, most importantly, administration of Haldol, was discontinued.

I shared my concerns with the hospitalist and asked specific questions about the edema (swelling) in his legs, lethargy and slurring words and loss of appetite that I had observed. I also asked whether or not this cardiac episode was perhaps a side effect of his prescribed medications and or their interactions. He answered that it was very likely and that judging by his improvement with IV fluids, and perhaps some other interventions that I cannot recall, he was definitely doing better. The medication interactions were a problem, which was in agreement with my doctor friend's assessment.

I was so grateful that the nurse had sent my uncle to the hospital. I felt that now I could get some clear answers about his health, behavioral concerns and his prognosis. I called the nurse at his facility that night, to thank her directly for making the 911 call. I was hopeful that now we could find a better way to help my uncle. I felt vindicated and validated and most of all extremely grateful to the night nurse for her honestly and willingness to stick her neck out and do what was best for my uncle, not what may have been in line with facility politics and expectations. She was very pleased to be acknowledged.

I am not saying that the facility was all bad, or that all staff were incompetent. Within all institutions there is a system in place. With each of my five experiences I saw how each system was different, yet also the same in many respects. The one theme that ran through all of them was that as a caregiver, I found it essential to try first work to with and within the system i.e. learn the system as best as possible, find the right people to talk to or reach out to for help within that system. However, sometimes I needed to go around or outside of the internal system to get help, answers, or relief. It is not always easy to do, but in the end it is well worth the time, risk and effort.

It turned out that my uncle's heart disease was at a critical level and that open-heart surgery was an option, but the risks far outweighed the benefits. The doctor laid out all of our options but did not tell me what I should choose. The surgery would be risky due to his overall health condition, which included very brittle diabetes, so healing could be jeopardized.

I asked multiple questions before asking, "Would my uncle be best served through hospice care at this point?" Because my uncle had qualified for hospice care while still in Michigan, I thought that my request was not off base. I also knew in my heart, that he was not going to get better. His behaviors could not be managed, due to his advancing dementia and his health issues were not going to be "cured." He was in pain emotionally and physically and I knew that no matter how many drugs they gave him this was not the answer.

Hope, Hospitalist, Hospice

After he conferred with the cardiologist, the hospitalist felt that hospice was an appropriate option to consider. The hospitalist contacted the hospice center. That afternoon I met with the hospice intake worker. The plan was that once my uncle was discharged back to the memory unit in the facility, the hospice nurse would provide services there and we would finalize all the paperwork at this time.

My uncle needed to stay a few more days in the hospital, and I visited him every day to make sure he was getting his basic needs met and to keep him company. On one of my visits, I found out that the hospitalist was a great golfer, who enjoyed talking to my uncle and as you might guess, my uncle was thrilled about swapping stories. I could not have asked for a better match for my uncle. He came back to being himself again, without the fog of the many medications they had him on in the memory unit.

I met that afternoon with the hospice care and they concurred that he qualified for their services. From my prior experiences I felt relief. I knew his care in the Memory Unit would be overseen by their frequent visits and that his medications would be changed and only the ones that were considered palliative would be maintained. I was optimistic that the right decision was made and had heard great things about the Hospice Care that had taken my uncle's case. The director of nursing at the facility raved about the hospice liaison, who had worked with them for years and they had nothing but great results with her. I was to meet her before my uncle was discharged. Unfortunately, what was presented ended up becoming untrue two days after my uncle's admission to hospice care.

Because of my prior experience with the facility doctor, I asked if the hospice physician could manage my uncle's care, and I was told this was feasible. My primary concern was that someone other than the facility doctor, whom we had issues with, would oversee his medications. I did not realize that this was not a popular request and that I was doing something against protocol. I was at this point having some deep doubts about my request and questioned myself. On the other hand, my gut told me I was doing the right thing. Turns out the hospice doctor did not want to do this, which only acted to make me doubt my request more.

While I was going back and forth in my mind, I ran into a woman whom I knew, whose mother lived in the facility where my uncle was. We saw one another going in and out periodically and would chat. As had happened before, I had another chance encounter with this woman and she asked me how my uncle was doing, I told her about his trip to the hospital and the medication reactions. I also shared that I had difficulty with the facility doctor. She pulled me closer and said, "That Doctor nearly killed my mother with the medications he put her on." She went on to say that she, "never would let her mother see him again."

The story she told me was timely and helpful, in that, it strengthened my convictions to stick with my request to have the hospice doctor be the attending physician for my uncle. I knew my uncle was very vulnerable and at risk. I wanted the best oversight of his care, and this woman's story solidified that I had a right to ask for the hospice physician and I was ultimately successful. Despite getting over this hurdle, I ran into more problems with the hospice agency services and staff members.

Unfortunate Circumstances, Communication Breakdown, Critical Needs

Long story short, the assigned hospice nurse, whom everyone loved and told me was the best and most attentive nurse they knew, stopped showing up and never contacted me. We had one intake/orientation interview, that went fairly well, but in retrospect, she seemed distracted and evasive when I asked questions. At the end, she did indicate that someone else would fill in for her the following week, but she would be back. Unfortunately, she never came back and the temporary nurse assigned was overwhelmed with cases and was also not showing up the days that had been assigned. When I finally reached the temporary nurse, she knew nothing about my uncle's history.

I decided to call the hospice social worker, who I met during the admissions process for help. She became my "go to" contact and helped me immensely from this point forward. However, despite her help, I continued to have problems with this hospice service and spent countless hours, trying to help my uncle get the care he deserved and needed. At this point, the facility and the hospice care were not communicating well either.

We had a critical medical need that required specialized attention, because, my uncle had developed a serious foot ulcer and being diabetic it required monitoring and specialty wound care. The social worker was very accommodating over the phone but I still saw big gaps in communication between my uncle's facility, and the hospice nurses. I continued to get vague answers regarding what happened to the nurse we were assigned to in the first place and the continuity of care was nonexistent. Because of my prior experiences, I knew that this was not normal, and was detrimentally affecting my uncle's quality of care.

The final straw was an encounter with a hospice nurse dispatched on the weekend based upon my call for help. My uncle's foot wound was causing him tremendous pain. When she came she was agitated and made derogatory comments to me in front of my uncle. She did not feel that the call was warranted. The fact was the nurse did not show up that week because of the shortage in staff. This nurse was rude and determined that the wound was a diabetic ulcer and left. This is when I decided that I needed to meet with the "powers that be" to address the problem of the missing hospice nurse. I also called the hospice center and complained about the nurse's behavior during her visit with my uncle over the weekend. After this episode I knew that I had to do something to protect my uncle's well-being. The wound was very serious and needed more medical attention as soon as possible. I understood it could not be cured, but the point was that the management of his pain was ineffective due to inconsistent care and attention.

Requesting a Meeting

In hopes to improve the communication between the hospice staff and the facility, I went directly to the facility director's office and also called the hospice social worker to ask for a meeting. I asked that the hospice staff, the memory unit staff and the director of nursing attend in hopes that together they could develop a plan of action to address the gap in hospice care since the nurse assigned left unexpectedly. And, I was open to anyone else they felt should be there. At this point, nobody seemed to know if the assigned nurse was returning to work or not. Without an assigned hospice nurse in place the continuity of nursing care had come unraveled. The end result was poor care coupled with poor follow up on the part of the facility and the hospice agency.

As caregiver, feeling very responsible for my uncle's comfort, I was feeling extremely frustrated, because I felt that I was being given the run around. Fortunately, the social worker had been responsive each time I had called her and she was very supportive of my request to bring all parties together in the same room at the same time. She agreed that the communication between the facility and the hospice care was disjointed and territorial. Not my problem specifically, but it effected the care of my uncle and I needed to assertively ask how this situation was going to be rectified.

The temporary hospice nurse assigned to the case came to the meeting late, but I was still happy to see she showed up at all. What I learned was that this nurse was not going to continue as my uncle's hospice care nurse. Regardless of this, the staff thought it best to have her there to pass along recommendations and information to the nurse that would ultimately be assigned to the case.

I would love to say this one meeting took care of everything, but it didn't. What it did achieve was improvement in communication, and permitted me to express my valid concerns and connected me with a contact person for each of my concerns. And, most significantly, this meeting raised vital awareness for those who were in supervisory roles, as to their system breakdown.

Of all my hospice experiences this was the worst, except for the social worker on the case. In a larger city, there would have been more hospice options to choose from. In my case, this was the only agency in the area, so I had to work with what was there. It took time and emotional energy but in the end it was worth the effort.

Although the original assigned nurse never returned, my uncle was assigned one primary hospice nurse after about a month. The primary need became treatment of his foot wound. If it could not be properly treated, he would have to be moved to a nursing home, which would have been the worst thing for my uncle. The wound nurse turned out to be excellent and she stayed in contact with me and developed a consistent and caring rapport with my uncle. Without my intervention, I know that my uncle's needs would have fallen through the cracks.

What I learned here was that although dealing with multiple systems is intimidating, if and when you know that someone you care for, is not getting proper or consistent care while in hospice care follow your gut. Start by asking questions and go to directors and supervisors to see if they can help. If individual meetings don't bring results, then ask for a team meeting with all relevant parties. If you do not live nearby to attend, ask for a teleconference.

My Uncle Dies with Care and Comfort

Within about a six to eight weeks under hospice care my uncle passed peacefully. I knew more of what to expect, but that didn't take away the pain of the loss. I was there with the hospice nurse and my uncle when I went to say my final goodbye. He knew I was there, and he knew that I was going to a conference for the Institute for the Ages. I told him exactly when I was leaving and what day I would return. When I told the nurse at the desk I was leaving she told me not to worry, that there was nothing more I could do. I called in the morning and he was still breathing, and sleeping comfortably. Within an hour of my call my uncle died. The nurse called me immediately to tell me that he had passed. I asked whether anyone was with him when he died. The facility nurse, one whom I trusted and respected, had just checked on him and saw he was sleeping. She returned in ten minutes and he was gone. Ironically, I was just leaving my driveway with my husband to go to the conference. I cried, but felt a sense of relief for my uncle, whom I knew had been miserable for a very long time.

Reflections on the Importance of Oversight

This hospice experience was much rockier than my others, but if it taught me one thing, it was to persevere when you know in your heart that the service your loved one is receiving is deficient. If you need someone to assist you in the process there are choices. One being: Caregiver Action Network. http://caregiveraction.org. This is one of many sites that can be found on the Internet for caregivers providing useful information, resources and support.

Friends and family are, of course, always an option for support if you cannot do it alone. Attending meetings alone can be intimidating, so asking or needing help is nothing to feel embarrassed about. I have had friends tell me how they "fell apart," or cried and could not talk during a meeting requesting information about a care concern for their loved one. They became so upset they had to leave before anything was settled. Local services can also be found if you need someone to attend meetings with you. The process is difficult at times, but it is part of the caregiver role and is certainly one of the most important parts of the "job."

Finally, my "near" distance, rather intensive, proactive four months of caregiving for my uncle, was oftentimes overwhelming, frustrating and sad, but I would not trade it for anything. He arrived in Florida at the end of October, 2013 and died in the first week of February, 2014. The time seemed much longer than it actually was. Most days were stressful. I felt tremendously responsible to ensure that my uncle's life was comfortable, stimulating and supportive of his needs. I could not always achieve this because of reasons that were not always within my control. I questioned myself often and tried not to be too hard on myself when things didn't go as I hoped or planned.

Moving my uncle to Florida was not easy and the care was not always up to what I felt it should be. It was not all bad and there were many positives about his having time with family. One thing I loved was listening to stories he told me that I had never heard, and taking him for walks to watch the golfers that played behind his facility. His decline in physical and mental health was quick. I cherish the times that he was lucid and conversant and able to enjoy life. We loved watching the Golf Channel together and he even still gave me tips on my golf swing. When he was at his best, the staff loved him. These are the memories I hold onto.

CHAPTER FIFTEEN

MY BROTHER'S STORY

Once again, one phone call launched me into another, yet different, long distance caregiving role. On July 19, 2010, my older brother's world was turned upside down when he was suddenly diagnosed with colorectal cancer at age fifty-eight. He had never been married, had no children, and at the time did not have a girlfriend. It was quickly evident he needed family support. Simply writing the series of events associated with my brother's diagnosis, subsequent medical complications, treatment and ultimate death was daunting for me. Keep in mind that this was also during the time I was caring for my aunt and uncle.

In the beginning, I had no idea how much support he would need, but because I had the flexibility to help if and when he needed it, I realized that I would be the one to assist in any way that I could. My prior experiences helped me know what to expect, but what it did not prepare me for, was a whole new set of circumstances and feelings that surrounded his medical, emotional and financial needs.

This Time Was Different

My brother and I had a very close relationship, which was just one of the reasons this time was different. The fact that he was still young seemed that much more critical and magnified my feelings. I felt guilty that my life was going well, while he faced cancer among other issues. This feeling hovered over me the entire time I cared for him, like a bad dream, from which I couldn't wake up. What I was not anticipating at the time was that soon after his cancer diagnosis, he had a life threatening brainbleed, which created a situation filled with extenuating circumstances and hurdles that I could never have anticipated. In order to survive the demands of juggling my life, my aunt and uncle's, and now my brother's meant that I had to prioritize to whom I would devote my time, based upon who needed me the most at any given time. I learned once again to give some of this responsibility to others, who were willing and able to help, but as before, these decisions came with their own set of issues.

For six long months, my brother fought for his life. Together we rode a roller coaster of events, emotions and challenges that were stressful, intense and unpredictable. I know the ride was much worse for him than for me; however, I felt every bump, derailment and scary feeling that comes with being out of control and knowing that there is a potential for a fatal crash ahead. Whenever I had fun during these six months of caregiving, I felt tremendously guilty, which lessened my joy. In the pages that follow, I discuss what it was like to take on a caregiving role for my older brother and why this time was so difficult and how it ended up taking its toll on me.

Because this was now my fifth time in ten years with five different familial relationships and personalities, along with differing medical, mental and aging concerns, I learned many new ways to manage not just one long distance caregiving situation, but more than one at the same time. One of the biggest lessons learned was that I no longer could continue helping my family without addressing my own feelings and needs. I didn't have time for traditional therapy or a support group. My schedule was unpredictable, and I was travelling most weeks, so through some luck and outreach on my part, I was able to get help through a Life Coach. Later I will explain how this came to be and how it was a practical way for me to receive professional support.

My Feelings Were Different

My brother needed to be a part of the process of managing his own care, whenever and wherever possible. I knew that there were times that I had to help him and wanted to, but my feelings oftentimes overwhelmed me and sometimes upset him. This was true with my other experiences, but this time my feelings were beyond anything I had yet experienced. People would admire what I was doing, but all I thought was that my help was falling short and that I was powerless in truly making a difference by changing the course of my brother's recovery.

I knew that many people survive cancer, and I tried to be optimistic and hopeful, but for some reason I was deeply concerned from the get go. I had a bad feeling about what lay ahead for him and I could not shake it.

In retrospect, I believe that some of my brother's feelings were much the same. Being so close all of our lives, I could not help but identify strongly with his situation.

Together, my brother and I worked at positive thinking and a fighting spirit, but our pessimism lurked beneath the surface at all times. Watching him face the challenges of cancer and the serious effects of an extenuating medical crisis before his treatment began, took its toll on me emotionally and physically. I wanted the diagnosis to be a mistake, and I wanted to hear that his cancer was found at a treatable, early stage. I also wanted him to be the brother I had before all of his health problems began. His life changed in an instant, and it seemed like we never were able to catch our breath.

The common question asked by my brother of, "why me," was to be expected. What wasn't expected was what my own reactions and feelings would be to his feelings and needs. I had a hard time coping with his anger, sadness and sometimes just the look on his face made me want to cry. I admit that there were times that I wanted to be anywhere else than with him. Not because I didn't want to be there to support him, but because of how hard it was to hear his anguish, see his pain and watch him suffer.

His anger became my biggest challenge. What was most difficult for me was when I was the target of his pain, frustration and rage. Some days it was more than I could bear; other days, I seemed better able to be the whipping post for his feelings of helplessness and fear. I always understood that what he was going through was extremely difficult, and I understood why he felt angry, but my reactions resulted in physical fatigue and often a feeling of being trapped. To top it off, my feelings got in the way of being able to help him more effectively than I could. Having such feelings felt heartless and I beat myself up for having them. I knew that I wasn't alone, and often expressed the fact that there were others with even more difficult challenges in the world, and told myself not to complain, but still felt badly most days.

It wasn't doom and gloom all of the time; there were good days and bad days, as one would expect. He often expressed feeling grateful for me being there to help him, and expressed optimism and a strong will to live. Unfortunately, I did not always share his optimism. I never let him know this, but it was the demon in my own mind that continued to nudge me every so often, making me feel awful for thinking negatively. Prayers of hope kept me going.

Adapting To Our New Roles

My brother was four years older than I, and as with most sibling relationships, being older, he taught me a lot growing up and felt it was his
place to look out for me. And, as many brothers and sisters do, I also looked
out for him. Despite these established lifelong roles, when I took on a caregiving position, whatever balance and rhythm we had in our relationship
was turned on its head. One issue in the mix was feeling that some of my
brother's life decisions contributed to his current health situation. Not that
I thought that he caused his cancer, but perhaps the choices he had made
may have played a role in how things ended up in the long-run. Thoughts
like, why didn't he get the colonoscopy that his doctor had recommended
two or three times over the prior few years? Why didn't he accept my offer
to help pay for some of the expense of a colonoscopy, if not all of it? Such
thoughts were put aside as I talked myself out of blaming him and made
the decision to do anything that I could to help him. It took energy to stay
focused.

Changing Communications

My brother's new found need for my help meant we needed to have
frequent phone calls about subjects that neither he nor I wanted to talk
about nor did we ever imagine that we'd be faced with dealing with such
concerns together. An example of our difficulty with our new roles came
through loud and clear in our communications soon after we learned of his
cancer diagnosis. Our calls centered on my attempts to support him, not
only emotionally but in managing all of his affairs, which included basic
things like bill payments, applications for assistance, shutting off services
such as cable; the list went on. It was understandably difficult for him to be
suddenly dependent upon me. We both felt out of control of the situation
and as a result, our conversations sometimes became heated.

I recall one such time when he called me around my bedtime. I left the
bedroom to talk in the kitchen. I stood at the sink, listening to him express
his fears and trying desperately to somehow ease his anxiety and stress, but
my words felt empty and meaningless. He was stressing over the appointments that had been set up and wondering how he was going to handle his
life. He was angry and his rage on the other end of the line was very difficult
to hear. My heart ached for what he must have been feeling yet this time

and other times ahead, I wasn't always as patient as I thought I should be with him. He wanted answers from me that I could not produce. During these calls I felt like nothing I said was helpful. I remember during more than one conversation, wanting to hang up on him to put an end to the exhausting loop, which seemed to be never ending.

My way out was to tell him that I had to get back to whatever I was doing and/or get my rest, if he called late at night. I promised that I would be there for him every step of the way. I followed up with assuring him that I would help him get done what needed to be done and help with whatever he couldn't do at the time. Throughout his care such calls between us continued. Once he was in the hospital then the nursing home, his calls would very often come in the middle of the night or very early in the morning. I dreaded hearing the phone rang at such times, knowing that the call would not be easy. He had issues with the care he was receiving and was in unmanageable pain. He would call to tell me that he was not getting help from the staff on duty. Such calls meant that I would have to take action the next day, or that night. What I realize now is that such conversations and our ability to communicate honestly became pivotal to my being able to be an effective advocate for him.

When It All Began

The diagnosis of cancer seemed sudden and unexpected, but in retrospect there were clues that he was having some health concerns based upon things he told me going as far back as the summer before the diagnosis. Once he began sharing some symptoms he was having and what the doctor had told him, I became concerned. For most of the year, he and I lived in different states. He shared his worries about his digestive health the summer before while we were both in Michigan. He also came to Florida in the spring to stay for a month or two to work on his art. This particular year, he went back to working on music, his other talent. He had previously put his music career on hold, while he started painting and selling his beautiful oil paintings. Now he was motivated to write songs again. His ultimate goal was to produce a CD of songs and he worked night and day to get it completed.

As he worked on this endeavor, he rented a place about two miles from our home. While he was there, we enjoyed spending time together and golfing; something that we had in common and both loved. During this time, he began complaining about feeling weak when we golfed. I attributed his complaints to his tendency to be very hard on himself. He was a perfectionist. He wanted to hit the ball purely and with distance. He was adamant that something was wrong with him and that was why he wasn't playing well. We had our typical sibling rivalry. I thought he was being dramatic and told him he was playing well, not to worry and just enjoy the beautiful day and our time together. I wasn't ready to hear that he was ill.

I had a nagging feeling that maybe there was something wrong with him. He continued to have other symptoms and concerns. What came back to me was that at the end of the prior summer, he shared some symptoms he was having and I remembered telling him to get a colonoscopy based on what he told me. Another clue that something wasn't right was that I had asked him a number of times to go on a bike ride with me but he kept declining, which was not like him. Finally, on one of his last days with us, I convinced him to go for a ride with me before he left for Michigan. During the ride he complained of pain and told me he was going to go to an urgent care center as soon as he could. I agreed that this was a good plan. He never ended up going before he left Florida. He decided it best to wait to see his doctor in Michigan.

The day he was leaving to drive back to Michigan, my husband and I met him to have breakfast together to say goodbye. When we were finished he asked me to come out to his car to talk. It was then that he turned to me and said, "There is something really wrong with me." I pleaded with him to see a doctor as soon as he got home, and most importantly to get a colonoscopy. Just the year before this, our first cousin had been diagnosed with Stage III colon cancer, which put my brother at a higher risk. I was adamant that he get the colonoscopy when he got home.

No Health Insurance Coverage

One reason he was slow to act on his symptoms was due to his lack of health insurance. He did not qualify for assistance and basically fell through the cracks due to the cost of insurance. He was able to obtain county insurance that afforded him access to outpatient care only. This was important and helpful to him because he was diagnosed with depression and bi-polar disorder for which he took medication and was followed by a psychiatrist on an outpatient basis. Colonoscopy screenings or hospitalizations were not covered. I suggested that he go get it scheduled and find out the cost with an adjusted fee based upon a "sliding scale" determined by income and ability to pay. I told him that we would pick up what he couldn't afford.

Once he got back home he did go to his doctor. During his exam the doctor found a cyst that needed to be removed and biopsied. The cyst had nothing to do with his digestive symptoms and was thankfully benign. However, my brother shared that for the past three years his annual fecal tests indicated a need for a colonoscopy. Now I was really worried and upset that he had never gotten one done. Once he healed from this cyst removal, the doctor told him that he would be ready to have the colonoscopy. It was scheduled for July nineteenth, which coincidentally was scheduled on the same day my sister was to fly into Michigan for her summer visit.

Family Dynamics...Who's going to Help My Brother?

Despite the positive results of the cyst biopsy, he remained very anxious about his health. He called and begged me to come down to drive him for his colonoscopy. This was not a good time for me to help due to some commitments I had, so I offered to call our nephew, who lived near him. My nephew was initially resistant to helping, because he was understandably stressed by the fact that soon he and his family would be moving to Wyoming. He had a lot to take care of and he didn't think he would have the time. I called my sister to ask that she please encourage her son to help his uncle, our brother, by driving him to the colonoscopy. He would not commit to doing it because of the fact that he had to watch his youngest child. This created some family tension, but I decided to persist with my request.

At the same time my brother was asking that I be the person to take him. Once again I asked my nephew to please help his uncle out and again asked my sister to encourage him to do this. My nephew was not working because he had already left his job to prepare for moving. I admit that I was resistant to driving two-hundred plus miles to take him for his colonoscopy, but this was due to my feeling stressed by my aunt and uncle's situation. I wanted a break. This did not mean that I would not help, but I felt that another family member or friend, who was physically closer at the time, should step up to the plate. Thankfully, after quite a few phone calls, my nephew agreed to take him. On the same day, he also would be picking up my sister at the airport. The fact that these two things ended up on the same day turned out to be quite fortuitous considering the outcome of the colonoscopy.

Getting the Results

The plan was that my sister or my brother would call me to let me know the outcome. I carried my cell phone with me all day in anticipation of the call but by 4:00 p.m. I hadn't heard anything so called my sister. At "Hello," I immediately heard in her voice that something was wrong. She told me that the results of the colonoscopy were not good and handed the phone to my brother.

My brother's first words were, "It's not good. It's really bad." He repeated this a few times and then added, "I have rectal cancer, and the doctor said it is a rare type of tumor." My worst fear had been confirmed.

I felt badly for my sister, as this was supposed to be the first day of her vacation. During the time she was visiting Michigan, she and I spent most of our time together worrying and talking about our brother. I know that she, like me, had a very difficult time processing and accepting what he was facing. The one benefit was that we were all together as a family. The next step was for my brother to meet with a surgeon to learn what the treatment protocol would be, and more about the type of tumor and the prognosis. There was about a week in between this meeting and his meeting with the radiologist. In the meantime, my sister was next door to me, so we spent plenty of time together, worrying, talking and praying.

Meeting with the Surgeon

We were very fortunate that a relative of ours, a retired pathologist and professor, offered to review my brother's pathology report prior to our appointment with the surgeon. He explained to me that this was a very rare and difficult cancer to treat. He also kindly offered to review all of the pathology reports *pro bono*. His prognosis was not very promising. I did not share this with my brother. I felt that negative news coming from me would not be helpful. In addition, a gastroenterologist, who happened to be an acquaintance of mine and of my brother's, happened to golf in a group with me for the one and only time ever a few weeks before my brother had his colonoscopy. During the round she shared that she had done thousands of colonoscopies. After learning of my brother's diagnosis, I called her and told her about what was found and she kindly offered to listen in on the consult with the surgeon via speakerphone. She generously provided consultation time without charging, asking instead that we make a donation in an amount to a charity of her choice.

The help provided by both experts was fortunate and comforting for us, simply because we knew them personally. We could trust them, not just because of their many years of professional experience, but also because of their vested personal interest in my brother. Many of their answers were not what we wanted to hear, but they were certainly what we needed to hear in preparation for what might happen next. Their input gave us time to formulate our own questions before the meeting with the surgeon. As I have said before, "knowledge is power," especially in regard to health concerns and making informed decisions. The lesson of the importance of being proactive as caregivers was something I learned early on with my father. I offered to and wanted to accompany my brother for his appointment with the surgeon. This time I knew that I wanted to be there to help him no matter what my conflicts or commitments might be.

Help From an Old Friend

Another help for my brother and myself was that of a mutual friend of ours, Bob, who offered to come with us to the appointment with the surgeon. Bob had been a good friend of ours for many years. Having him there was very helpful. This experience confirmed that bringing a friend or family member into such an emotional meeting, who could help listen and take notes, was quite important. Not only did Bob accompany us to the meeting with the surgeon, he stayed the course and became an extremely helpful source of support for both my brother and myself. In retrospect, I know now that people other than family members can be a great source of assistance and should not be counted out, even if we have a difficult time with the personal nature of such situations.

What We Heard From the Surgeon

The recommendation by the surgeon was that the tumor needed to be reduced in size before any surgery could safely be done to remove it. He also explained more about the nature of the tumor, which was called a "Signet Ring Cell" tumor. What we heard was that it was extremely rare, and aggressive. Those words were tough to hear for everyone in the room. Our gastroenterologist friend asked questions over the speaker phone, which helped us to get more important information. To shrink the tumor my brother would need to undergo radiation treatments. Preparation for radiation required that he needed to be "tattooed" to map out the target area where the radiation should be directed. In addition he would receive oral chemotherapy. The treatment protocol meant that my brother's next step would be to meet with an Oncologist and a Radiologist, which the surgeon's office arranged.

Reality Was Setting In

Reality was setting in, and it was not easy. To say that all of this was devastating for my brother to hear is an understatement. We left the appointment with a dark cloud hanging over all of our heads. One thing that took the sting out of that morning was that my brother had just had his music burned on CD's. We listened to his new CD in the car and tried to block out our feelings and remain optimistic. After all, treatment was scheduled and we were looking ahead to preparation for surgery and removal of the cancerous tumor.

My brother understandably was stressing over the how's and why's of the whole process. He wondered about who would help him, about money, work, and how his daily life would be managed. Knowing that it was an aggressive and fast-growing type of tumor made all of us worry that much more. I learned that most signet ring cell carcinomas are not found early enough to treat effectively. As I write this, it is five years after the time of my brother's diagnosis, and my research indicates it remains a difficult type of tumor to find in its early stages, which directly impacts success of treatment and survival rates.

Treatment Plans Are Now In Place

His diagnosis and treatment plan came together in late July/early August of 2010. Getting the tattoos done was one step closer to treatment beginning. At the same time the oncologist was pushing him to agree to take an experimental chemotherapy drug to treat the tumor as part of research. We knew he needed chemotherapy, but he was expecting that this would be done with tried and true drugs; he was very resistant to this idea. He wanted to go with the standard protocol. I did not encourage him one way or the other, but asked him questions and listened to his concerns. I felt that this was truly his decision to make. Most importantly, I verbally committed to my brother that I would be there for him whenever he needed me. Unfortunately, before any radiation treatment actually began, an unexpected medical event occurred shortly after the tattooing procedure, which postponed the onset of any treatment, and drastically changed my brother's life.

Another Call, another Crisis

Shortly after his radiation tattooing had been completed, without warning, the need for me to drive down to help him came fast and furiously via a phone call. It was my husband's birthday, and in keeping with tradition, I made him a special breakfast. While relaxing afterwards an old friend of mine called. While we were talking on the phone, the call-waiting beeped in and interrupted our call. Because of the fact that I was still taking care of my aunt and uncle from afar, I always looked at my caller ID to see who was calling. I recognized the area code, but not the number. Although it was not a recognizable number to me, it was from my brother's area code, so I told my friend that I had go, and I'd call her back.

When I answered, the voice at the other end of the line said, "This is the emergency room of ... Hospital and we have a relative of Caroline Sheppard here with us in our emergency room." I was asked to confirm that I was my brother's sister and then I was told that my brother had experienced a "brainbleed." The person on the other end of the line further said, "Your brother drove himself here and is being admitted to the Neuro ICU (Intensive Care Unit).

As is standard procedure, the person on the other end of the line minimized the potential effects of the bleed and any expected future problems. I was told that they expected, "The bleed would resolve itself within a few days and that he should be discharged within three or four days or so." The ER nurse added that it was "surprising" that he was able to drive to the hospital without a problem. She said that he was, "Very lucky to have made it without having an accident."

Despite hearing that he had made it successfully and safely to the hospital, my initial reaction was shock. My second reaction was to try to stay calm and ask as many questions as I could. I prayed for it not to be too serious and that he would not have any negative residual side effects. I recall physically shaking. I asked what was meant by a "brainbleed?" She did talk in vague terms about a possible stroke and that they would know more when the CT scans, etc. came back.

A clue that this was serious was that it was strongly suggested that I come to the hospital as soon as possible. I could not realistically get there for about five hours due to the distance between where I lived and where the hospital was located. The best option was for me to send my nephew, who lived near the hospital. What I realized immediately was that I was facing another logistical challenge as a caregiver, and I could not believe it was happening again. I was trying to process all that the ER staff member had told me and felt completely overwhelmed. I recall wanting to know much more than what she had already told me, so I asked more questions such as what symptoms my brother was having. The nurse explained that he had "a sudden onset of a severe headache, which awakened him in the early morning hours." He reportedly realized that he needed help.

Rather than call 911, which would have been the best plan, my brother drove himself to the hospital, so that he would not be taken by ambulance to the county hospital. Driving himself was typically not the best choice, but in this case it ended up being a good thing. Turns out that by driving himself he went to the same hospital he had been to the week before for his radiation preparation appointment. The most positive outcome of this decision was that he had just days before filled out all the emergency contact information. My brother put me down as the contact person, which is why the ER knew how to call me. I remember feeling that although this all seemed really bad, I was grateful for the serendipitous events that seemed to have protected my brother from having an accident, or delaying him from getting help as soon as he did. This gave me a sense of hope that things would be okay.

Another lucky event was the morning this happened it was in the summer on a Sunday. My brother lived in a busy college town, where traffic is typically very heavy during a normal weekday or on a football Saturday. Being a Sunday at about five in the morning, nobody was on the road, which seemed to be "nothing short of a miracle." I was about two hundred miles away from him at the time of the call and to get there required some travel challenges. It was a matter of my riding my bike over three miles to take a ferry to get my car and then drive four hours. I told the nurse that I wouldn't be there before early evening. She assured me that my nephew coming to the hospital until I could get there would be okay.

Sharing the News

Before I could make any firm plans, I had to tell my husband about the call and that I had to leave ASAP. My husband's birthday was abruptly interrupted by yet another one of my family members' need. I think that by this time he was getting used to it. Nonetheless, I was dreading having to tell him about the call and that I had to leave. He had always been supportive, but this time I wasn't sure he would understand or how he'd react.

I took a deep breath and went to tell him about my brother's brainbleed and that the nurse wanted me to come right away. My husband was a bit confused at first, because the phone had never actually rung. The last he knew I was speaking to my friend. Next thing he hears from me is that I need to leave to go be with my brother. Fortunately, as in every other circumstance, he was helpful and supportive. His acceptance of my leaving made a huge difference for me. It's hard enough to leave when you yourself do not want to go, but add someone fighting your need to help a family member in need, and it makes a bad situation worse.

This crisis felt different than anything I had yet to experience with my parents and my aunt and uncle. Despite the knowledge I had gained along the way, this one kicked me in the gut. The brainbleed, along with his cancer diagnosis, added a whole new dimension and layer of stress and challenges that I did not feel ready to meet.

Calling My Nephew

I prioritized those I needed to inform. After telling my husband, I called my nephew, who lived near my brother and asked him to please go be with his uncle at the hospital and that I would be down in about five hours. This is the same nephew who had driven my brother for his colonoscopy a few weeks before. He was as shocked as I was as I tried to tell him the news as gently as possible and also assure him that I would get there as soon as humanly possible. Come to find out, the night before this fateful morning, my brother had dinner with our nephew and family to say goodbye. We have a great picture of my brother with our nephew, his wife and our great niece and nephew. So the news of his brain hemorrhage seemed even more surprising to all of us. Even though we knew he was just diagnosed with cancer, this event seemed to come out of the blue. We had even commented that my brother looked great in the photo they had sent via email the night before. I remember thinking that he didn't look sick at all.

Calling My Sister

I needed to call my sister, but decided to wait until I got in my car where I knew I would have time to talk without interruption. It was a Sunday morning and she would be conducting services where she lived in a Mountain Time zone, two hours earlier than my time. Once I was on the expressway and knew that her services were finished, I called. As I shared what had happened I could hear her sadness come through loud and clear. She, like me, could not believe this was happening. We both speculated about what could have caused the brainbleed. We wondered if it was the stress from his diagnosis and the plans and worry about how he would pay for his medical care, or that maybe his cancer had spread to his brain. We wanted an answer, which I understand was our attempt to gain some feeling of control over a circumstance that we had absolutely no power over.

It is true that just prior to the brainbleed, my brother was stressing over everything. He was worried about not having health insurance, money issues, not working; the list went on. He was angry at the world, and I couldn't blame him. One thing I knew he wanted was for me to be able to come down to help him more than I could at this point. It seemed that he could handle getting to and from the radiation treatments and if he needed a ride he had local friends who could help him out. If that didn't work, we'd "cross that bridge when we got there." With a guilty conscience, I knew that the bridge was here and even though I knew that I had no control of anything that had happened, I couldn't shake that nagging feeling again that maybe I should have or could have done something differently.

Arriving At the Hospital

When I arrived at the hospital, my nephew was there to greet me in the lobby. His facial expression, pale complexion and apparent exhaustion spoke volumes. As we took the elevator up to where my brother was in the Neuro ICU my stomach was in knots, and I had a sense of doom. The cancer diagnosis was bad enough, but now my brother was in a Neurological Intensive Care Unit with a brainbleed, something I knew very little about. As we walked by a waiting room we saw families huddled together, some praying, some sitting in silence. I imagined that they were waiting to hear news from a doctor or simply comforting one another while their loved one or friend lay in the ICU where all patients had some kind of head trauma, brain injury or brain-related disease requiring round-the-clock intensive specialty care.

Not knowing what to expect made me that much more anxious. Questions like what would he look like, would he know me went through my head. I found myself wanting to get to him as quickly as possible, but at the same time not wanting to be there at all. The reality of what lay ahead was becoming more real with every single step I took. As we approached the final corner of the long hallway, the nurses' station with multiple monitors was to my right. I stopped at the desk to announce that I was there for my brother. They told me to go see him first and then to stop and sign some paperwork. I asked a few questions and I was told he was stable and that they were monitoring his vitals 24/7. That was when I noticed the screen that showed him in his bed with his vitals in clear view behind their desk.

My nephew showed me to my brother's room. His bed was elevated facing the door, so as I entered he saw me right away. His eyes were half open, and what I clearly remember was that he looked so small and scared in the large hospital bed. He smiled very slightly right away, raised his hand and said, "Hi, Lin!" Hearing his voice, although a bit weak, and knowing that he knew who I was, was so comforting. I tried to be strong and reassuring on the outside, but inside I felt ill. I had a bad feeling about what this could mean in relationship to the start of his cancer treatment.

Being that it was a Sunday night and he was considered to be in stable but critical condition, I was given some basic information by the nurse on duty, but would have to wait until the next day to speak to the neurologist. During my initial phone call from the Emergency Room, it was suggested that my brother would only be in the hospital for about three or four days for monitoring and assessment. They explained that this type of, "brain-bleed," generally resolves itself. After it was determined that the bleed had stopped, and he was stable, he could go home. Sadly, this prognosis and projection was not accurate.

My nephew's wife and kids were scheduled to leave ahead of him the next day and he was to follow a few days later after completing the packing and meeting the moving van. The fact that he was not leaving with them was more than fortunate for me. I was able to stay with him for about three nights until we knew what the prognosis and treatment plan would be going forward. My goal was to stay for a short time and then go home for a few days and come back. My plans did not hold true.

Life Happens While We Make Other Plans

After what seemed like an eternity, the next day the neurologist visited my brother and then talked to me privately in the hall. He explained that the type of bleed was called a subarachnoid bleed, a type of stroke. I had planned to be there for three days but discovered that I would be there much longer. As time went on, I learned more and more about the potential and very real results of this type of brainbleed. I was told that brainbleeds often resolve themselves without any long-term effects. I was also told that there was a good chance that he could go home soon. The doctor did not think the brainbleed had any connection to his cancer. But, we were told that the radiation would need to be delayed until he was better. We did not know at this juncture how long this would be.

Brain Surgery Leads to Complications and More

My brother's brainbleed led to complications that were unforeseen and more than anyone could have imagined. The first complication was that fluid developed around his brain requiring emergency surgery to insert a shunt to drain the fluid. The shunt insertion had gone well, so I was really hoping to go back home soon to get organized and then come back. This idea was quickly thwarted by a complication with the shunt itself. Surgery always carries with it some a risk, but we were reassured that the procedure is not unusual and my brother should be fine after the fluid was removed from his brain.

Unfortunately, not long after the shunt was inserted, he developed a severe unrelenting headache, and a high fever from infection. Testing determined the infection to be ecoli, which had somehow entered his brain during or following the surgery. This news was frightening. I called my sister right away to tell her what was happening. His anticipated short-term stay in the ICU was no longer a reality. We had been so relieved after the successful shunt insertion and now this. We were told that the cause could have been from any contact with feces that entered the incision site. Nobody actually knew how it happened. He was given IV antibiotics and the shunt would remain in place, because removing it was a high risk as well.

Ultimately, my brother underwent three brain surgeries: First, there was fluid on the brain, which led to a shunt being placed into his skull to drain the fluid. Next, to handle the E Coli infection, which was a very serious and frightening development in his care and treatment. The third surgery was done to remove the shunt when the infection was cleared.

I was told by his neurologist not to leave until my brother was stabilized, which turned out be a very long twenty-three days. My husband, as he did many other times, was thankfully taking care of things at home. I had nothing scheduled that could not be cancelled or rescheduled. At the same time, my aunt and uncle's care needed oversight as well. I checked on them daily and stayed in touch with their facility when problems arose. My brother was my priority at this point.

Diminished Abilities

My brother had three brain surgeries in total within about one month's time. Each time the after effects were never easy. Lots of pain and diminished abilities increased each time. He was weak and had difficulty walking and had lost some of his skills, one very significant one being manual dexterity, which directly impacted his art ability and later we found out his guitar playing as well. This was devastating to watch. I hung onto hope that things would improve with therapy.

The end result, was that my brother's cognitive abilities were negatively affected, which led to testing by a neuropsychologist, who had been told by the therapeutic team that they noticed changes in his memory and abilities as did I. The neuropsychologist, who performed the testing, was excellent and was very kind in the presentation of his findings when he went over the results with me. The testing indicated that my brother was unable to handle his affairs and would be deemed incompetent and I would be the assigned guardian of his affairs. I was devastated by this news.

A brilliant artist and musician's life was changing right before my eyes and I had no power to stop what was happening to him. In my efforts to encourage him, I went and bought him the art pens and paper he wanted. These pens were the kind he used to illustrate my books. I could barely watch him as he struggled to draw a very simple picture. I could see his own despair and I tried to encourage him and focus on the positive of his trying. He never drew another picture after this one attempt. This was such a dark time.

My attempts to make everything better was normal. To try to diminish my own angst, I wanted to somehow make him feel better. As I write these words, I can still feel the uncomfortable feelings I had, but more importantly I remember feeling that my presence was sometimes a double-edged sword. The very reason that I was there was a constant reminder of the dependency my brother now had on me. Here was someone who, just a few months before, was capable of managing his own life, producing music and art and carrying on daily activities.

I hoped and prayed that his brain would find new pathways and that again he could again draw, paint, illustrate, write music and play instruments, sing and entertain others as he always had. I hung onto hope that his brain would heal and he'd be able to make critical and even daily life decisions again and I would be removed from this role. That time sadly never came. Fortunately, he retained his ability to speak and still could carry on great conversations. We even argued over politics as we always had. Unfortunately his judgement was impaired, and he was not able to drive or make major life decisions.

He continued to work hard in therapy. He was personable and the therapists liked him, which always helps. In the long run his physical health issues continued to overshadow everything and affected his progress. It was so discouraging. I tried to support him, in meaningful ways. I would be quiet when he wanted quiet, talk when he needed to talk, watch baseball when he wanted to watch baseball, talk politics when he wanted to talk politics, get him his favorite treats from the store, entertain him, or simply sit and watch him sleep, so that when he woke up, I'd be there for him. I wanted his treatments to work and I wanted him to be cured, but every new day, seemed to lead to another complication and another delay in treatment. All I could do was to try to make sure that he was receiving the attention and care that he deserved and needed.

After the surgeries and the infection, he became extremely weak. We were told that his radiation treatments could not begin until he was stronger physically. All this time, he stewed over the fact that he couldn't start his radiation, which meant he could not begin chemo treatments; the first essential piece in his fight against the aggressive rectal tumor. The clock was ticking. By this time, we were into September; the diagnosis of cancer happened back in July. One thing that continued to concern me was that the medical staff presented a vague and cautiously optimistic prognosis. In fact, the cancer had never been "staged" as being either Stage 1, 2, 3 or 4. To me this seemed unusual. I had known others who had cancer and they always seemed to know the stage. In my brother's case, the surgeon told us that it could not be determined until the surgery itself was performed. In retrospect, it was probably best we did not truly understand the poor odds for cure and survival of this type of tumor.

Moving To the "Step-Down" Unit-More Challenges Ahead

After being in the ICU for a total of twenty-three days, he was transferred to the hospital's "Step-Down Unit," where he would receive care that was less intensive, yet provided more individualized attention than a general inpatient floor. The transfer itself was easy and only required leaving ICU through a set of double doors and moving into a private room. This move was short in distance, but huge in boosting my brother's and all of our family's morale, because it meant that the treatment for his cancer could finally begin while he continued to recuperate. The delay of the onset of radiation and chemotherapy due to my brother's brainbleed and subsequent complications had been a big worry for my brother and our family. So hearing that he could begin treatment soon gave everyone hope. The plan was that after approximately two weeks in the Step-down Unit, he was to be transferred to a general patient floor for oncology care.

Unfortunately, our hopes were dashed when the care my brother received in this unit was not meeting his needs at many levels. The term, "Step-Down," took on a whole new meaning, in that, the quality of care was substandard and the response to concerns and needs were not responded to in a helpful or timely manner. My observation was that supervision and knowledge was lacking and was a surprising contrast to the wonderful care he received while in the ICU. He complained about the lack of attention and assistance he was receiving. When I tried to find someone to talk to about his concerns, I ran into dead ends and got the run around. Assurances and promises that were made by staff were not honored. Someone seemed to be dropping the ball, and my goal was to get to the bottom of things in order to improve my brother's situation. It was coming to a critical point, and his pleas to me for help were escalating.

Radiation Finally Begins

While still in the Step-Down Unit, his radiation treatment was finally scheduled. This, I found, was a "double edged sword!" The anxious feelings associated with waiting and worrying about the effects of the delay on my brother's treatment was now over with, yet the days ahead were filled with so many unknowns. I fortunately happened to be there one morning, when he told me that he had been told that he would be getting his first radiation treatment that day. Before we knew it, a gurney showed up outside his room. I went and asked some questions and found out that he would be going down for radiation within an hour or so, and they suggested that I accompany him.

Soon he was picked up and I anxiously followed along as he was wheeled in a bed down the halls to the elevators where he took one elevator for patients only, and I was sent on another and told to meet them at the radiation center in the basement of the hospital. Once there, I was told to follow the blue tape on the floor and meet them there. The trip down was lonely and unnerving. After getting off the elevator, I found myself overwhelmed with the amount of twists and turns in the basement halls that I had to take to get to the Radiation Department. It was a very long and lonely walk for me. I remember feeling that I needed to put on a good face for my brother and not tell him of my own worries. When we were reunited, he was very happy to see me. I could see the fear in his eyes. I tried to talk about benign subjects, like the baseball playoffs and other non-related things as he waited to be called in for his treatment.

The flow of patients being wheeled in for their treatment, made me think of an assembly line. One by one patients went in and came out. It was a depressing scene, but also gave me hope. I couldn't help but think of all of the people radiation had saved and hoped that this would be true for my brother, too. What we didn't know at this point, and were not told, was that the effects of the treatments for my brother could be especially bad because of where the tumor was located. The actual radiation treatment was not the problem in and of itself. The placement of the tumor was in a highly sensitive area and the radiation aggravated it intensely. Hence, the biggest issue was the excruciatingly painful side effects following each treatment. The pain became increasingly worse after each radiation. His bowels were completely messed up and any bathroom experience was racked with pain.

I remember trying to help him through these times and feeling completely helpless as I heard him cry out from his private bathroom.

Filing a Formal Complaint

Once the radiation began, the pain became intolerable. He told me that his Step-Down Unit night nurse was withholding his doses of pain medication. I had to find someone to talk to and asked first for a social worker. I had a private meeting with the social worker and explained my concerns. I had tried to find the Nurse Supervisor of the unit but was given the run around. Turned out that the supervisor was on sick leave and that there was nobody in place as yet to provide oversight of the unit. I decided after many issues and worry that my brother was not getting proper care that I needed to file a formal complaint. This ended up being another learning experience.

In this hospital, the name of the complaint department was "Excellence of Care." It seems every hospital has a different title for this service. I made an appointment to explain my concerns. I found that my concerns were valid. It turned out that the Stepdown Unit had undergone some unexpected staff departures and the supervisory nurse was on an unexpected leave.

I advocated for my brother and explained that one of my concerns was refusal by one particular night nurse to provide pain medication to him. She was simply resistant and was not following the treatment plan. He was only asking for the night dosage that was actually prescribed. Another issue was that he needed assistance to get to and from his bathroom and the aides were not responding to his bells. The nurses and aides on duty seemed overworked and had an attitude about my brother. I must add that most nurses were extremely kind and dedicated, but like anything in life, not everyone is good at what they do. It's the human condition, I suppose.

One memorable part of my encounter in the complaint department was the staff member I met with to explain my concerns. He began our meeting explaining to me that he suffered from "narcolepsy," and that he may fall asleep while we talked to one another. This is a neurological condition where individuals have no control over when they fall asleep. He did drift off a bit here and there but managed to get all of the relevant information related to my concerns. He took care of the situation, my brother's treatment improved and his pain medication was administered as it should be from this point forward. I was most afraid of retribution by the staff on the floor, but was assured that this would not happen. I had to trust the process and, thankfully, the complaint did the trick.

Aside from my proactive step to file a complaint, I followed up with the social worker, this time for me, as I needed to debrief and validate that what I did was the right thing. Filing the complaint was very distressing and although behind me, I was doubting my decision and worried about repercussions. I was only there for a few days at a time each week, and worried greatly about negligence occurring again. The social worker helped me to realize that it was healthy for me to bring in others to visit and be there for my brother whenever I went home. To ease my mind ahead of my leaving, I tried to anticipate potential needs that my brother may have while I was gone. Letting go was not easy. Having the social worker tell me that it was okay to leave and ask others to step in made a big difference for me. I admit I felt guilty but I also accepted that I needed a break and gave myself permission to do just that.

After two weeks in the Step-Down unit, my brother was moved to another wing of the hospital that had a general inpatient floor, with an emphasis on Oncology patients. His new room was state of the art and very accommodating, primarily because his room was private and spacious, with its own easy access, and large modern bathroom. We had no idea how long he would be staying in the hospital. As it turned out, he remained approximately fifty days. While there, he received three weeks of oral chemotherapy and thirty-one radiation treatments.

Five Wishes

When my brother first moved onto the Oncology floor, we were asked that he complete a form that spells out his wishes for end of life care, called "Five Wishes." He did not have a Living Will. Five Wishes was becoming a standard operating procedure for hospitals and nursing homes and the like, to clarify what type of care the patient wanted if they required life sustaining interventions or end of life care at any point in the patient's stay.

My brother and I initially attempted to complete the questionnaire together and found it extremely upsetting to both of us. For him the task was particularly sensitive, because he was not old, yet he was suddenly faced with outlining what his wishes would be if his cancer was incurable and death was near. His opinion was that he was going to survive; therefore, he need not complete the form. It was an emotionally charged exercise and one that he wanted nothing to do with and really resented my trying to help him.

I tried to explain that I wasn't giving up on him and that the hospital required that we complete the form but nothing seemed to help. This was one of those times I felt exasperated and one of my own wishes was to leave rather than argue with him anymore. On the other hand, I had been assigned as his guardian, so I had to do what I could to get the document completed for his file. For both of us, this was something new and, although I had helped my elderly relatives get their affairs in order, this was different.

Because of the sensitive nature of completing his five wishes together, I decided to reach out to another cousin, a Physician's Assistant, who lived nearby and also covered this hospital. I explained the situation to him and he offered to come help us get through the process. My cousin saved the day and came by to help us get through the form. Even with my cousin to help us, it was not easy to finish. One thing that helped was that I was my brother's guardian and I explained that if I were not there for some reason, and God forbid there was nothing for the hospital to follow, the choice would not be his choice. With spelling out his final wishes, he still had a voice and was part of the process. I could have left him out completely but didn't. That seemed to smooth the waters and we were able to move on.

CHAPTER SIXTEEN
THE FINAL MOVES

I had begun the process of applying for disability and Medicaid, all of which was slow and time consuming. I think what I learned most about this arduous process is that it is inefficient, frustrating and filled with waste. The application for disability was done over the phone with me sitting with my brother as he lay in the hospital bed answering questions he could answer. I would assist when needed, but remained sensitive not to answer anything I knew that he could handle himself. It was very important to give him agency wherever and whenever it was possible to do so.

Every day we waited for the Medicaid insurance to begin, meant that the hospital was housing my brother without medical insurance. The hospital had a private fund that supported patients such as my brother, while he waited for insurance support. It was limited in scope but was at least something for the hospital. I first asked about how his care would be covered when he was in the ICU. I sought out the social services department in the hospital and met with the financial aid people. I did this the morning after I arrived to see my brother after his brainbleed. This fund was established through donations and the hospital writing off some of their fees. It was not something that lasted forever.

Once he had been moved to the general oncology floor, the clock started ticking and the administration began to visit him every day and ask him what he was doing to get insured. Because I wasn't there at all times, this meant he was faced with these visits despite the fact that I had been assigned to manage his affairs. After each one of these visits, my brother would call me telling me that he was scared that they were going to "put him out on the street!"

These calls made me angry and I called the doctor to ask him to stop asking my brother about his insurance and that I was the one in charge of such things. The doctor was officious and came across as impatient with the situation. I assured him that I was in touch with Medicaid and that he did qualify and that the insurance was forthcoming. I also pleaded with him to talk to me, not my brother as his daily questioning was very stressful for him. I sought out the help of a hospital social worker again to provide support and advocacy, which did work to our advantage. I learned one more time, that to speak up in an assertive nonaggressive manner was the best way to get the help needed provided.

The issues surrounding getting insurance and dealing with the administrative red tape and hospital harassment made a difficult health situation that much more challenging, and this I know is something that did not just happen to me. Maybe your story isn't the same, but similar situations happen to people because of the systems themselves and the personalities involved. This theme ran through each one of my experiences at varying degrees of difficulty and with different parts of each system involved.

One built-in protection was that the hospital could not kick my brother out even though the hospital administrator wanted to, because at this time his opiate pain medication was administered through a port, which prevented him from being discharged, unless he were to go to a nursing home. Another thing in his favor was that he was in line to receive Medicaid. His condition and need for continued radiation treatments, which caused terrible side effects, along with his IV pain management helped to keep him in the hospital without insurance. Seemed like an odd thing to appreciate but priorities change in times like this.

In my brother's case, the hospital kept him far longer than they wanted to because of his pain medication needs. The oncologists still recommended chemotherapy; however, he was in such a weakened condition it was recommended that he be transferred to a nursing home (skilled nursing center) to build up his weight and strength so that he could withstand chemotherapy. We were all hopeful that this would go well and saw this as forward progress.

He could not be released until he was no longer dependent on a port to administer his opiate pain medications. We also needed to wait until he was found eligible for Medicaid, which was needed in order to pay for his nursing home care. Going home was not a consideration at this point in his care. Of course, my brother would have preferred going home, but he understood that he could not have managed his life alone and the hospital felt he needed twenty four hour supervision. When his Medicaid application was accepted, he was finally discharged from the hospital after a total of seventy-four days. We were all hopeful that the nursing home would be a move toward progress and health.

Unbearable Pain, Unrelenting Pain

Let me just say a bit more about the pain he experienced after leaving ICU. The pain he experienced after radiation was attributed to radiation side effects. He had cramping, severe diarrhea, backaches, and a persistent side ache on the left side of his back that seemed to migrate to other places. I bring this up to point out that it is important as a caregiver to know that it's okay to be persistent with our questions when whomever we are assisting is experiencing pain that does not seem to be helped by whatever intervention is being used.

After I would help him to and from the bathroom and back to bed he continued to writhe in excruciating pain. I personally felt his pain internally and I would re-experience these moments with flashbacks of what I heard and saw after I left him. The treatments took its toll on my brother in every way.

At one point he required a blood transfusion due to his low blood count as a treatment side effect, another sign that he was becoming weaker, which made me think he might not make it. I hated such thoughts, but they were not easy to suppress. My brother asked that I sit with him during his infusions, because they made him anxious. I did do this and hoped my sitting there was a good distraction for him. His anxiety increased with every new day; as did the pain medication. At this point a port was inserted so that he no longer received pain medication via intravenous injection to reduce the use of a needle.

In retrospect, I recall that during all of the time that my brother's pain kept escalating in the hospital, I had a gut feeling that there was something beyond the radiation that caused his back and hip pain. Back when he went for his first brain surgery his hip and back were causing him severe pain. His symptoms were addressed with opiate pain medication in the hospital; however, I cannot recall that any further testing was ever done to determine from where his back and hip pain was emanating. I recall that the answer was always associated with his radiation. I don't believe I ever explained that the back and hip pain was present prior to any radiation.

I do recall asking questions of the oncologist's Physician's Assistant and was given vague and evasive answers. I could not shake my feeling that something else was going on with his pain. I recall attributing his pain to sciatica like I myself had and I would massage his back for him whenever he complained. I figured that lying in bed a lot may have been at the root of the pain. No matter what interventions were tried, his back and hip pain continued. I did tell the nurses about his pain and the response was to medicate, not to investigate.

As you can imagine, this was frustrating and at times made me think that I was overreacting. He was on intravenous pain medication and the breakthrough pain was still frequent and unbearable. What this was, nobody would or could tell me. I believe now that the oncologist did know what his pain might have indicated. Why they did not do further tests to determine the source of such pain would only be a guess, but I believe it was related to his lack of insurance.

Discharge from the Hospital and Transfer to the Nursing Home

I would like to say that the move from the hospital to the nursing home went smoothly, but this was far from the case. Our first and biggest problem was that the social worker and discharge planner could not find a nursing home bed in the area near the hospital, which would be near his apartment as well. It took longer than expected to find a "bed" for him, so this meant more time in the hospital. After much worry for all of us, a bed was found in a town about one hour from his oncology treatment center, and his apartment. This presented some concerns, but there was absolutely no choice in the matter.

My sister and I wondered about travel logistics for anyone wanting to visit him. This worry was put to rest once we discovered that it actually was between two connecting airports and the drive was not difficult at all from either one. What I figured out, was that I could fly into the connecting airport in his home town, and use my brother's car. This move to what seemed like the middle of nowhere ended up having more than one benefit. Something we never could have anticipated or imagined at this point. Before I go into this, I need to explain the difficulties of the actual transfer from hospital to nursing home.

When it came to transfers from hospitals to nursing homes. I had learned a lot about the process from my helping my father, mother and aunt up to this point. I thought I had seen everything, and I was sorely wrong. I knew more of what to expect regarding the process, but what I could not have predicted was how well my brother would adjust to the nursing home. Nor could I predict how good the facility would be and if it would be a good fit for him. What I was more prepared for this time was the logistics; what was needed, who to talk to for assistance, and basically how to "work the system" when necessary. Despite my prior knowledge, the move from the hospital, starting with a long drive, which in and of itself was hard on my brother, did not go easily right from the start. I like to think that some of my work with children paid off in how I handled the first week of my brother's move to the nursing home, because it was an emotional roller coaster ride for sure.

The first problem centered on the fact that my brother's port to administer long term and very strong opiate pain medication was removed the day he was discharged from the hospital. What this meant was that this change in medication from IV to oral needed to be done carefully and with planning and forethought. I found out quickly that someone "dropped the ball" on sharing information and most importantly placing a timely prescription order for a change to oral medication in time for the nursing home to fill the order before my brother arrived.

Everyone knew the date in advance of when he would be discharged and transferred to the nursing home, yet when we arrived at the facility, his medication needs and orders had been mismanaged. The only solution was to find an alternative medication until the correct order came through, which ultimately did not happen until the next day. I vividly remember that my brother's pain became unbearable. He was having withdrawal reactions. The nurse on duty attempted to get things squared away, but it was evening and deliveries were done for that day. This was serious and clearly negligence as I saw it at the time. Mistakes can and do happen and this is why I am such a proponent of making sure that someone, who is not part of the system, be a watchdog in some capacity when someone cannot advocate for themselves.

I became an advocate in overdrive that first night. And, the situation only got worse. At this point, he was in a high level of distress. Times like these really tested my patience, faith and trust with those caring for my brother. I was determined to get the attention of the powers that be and thankfully with perseverance, proactive advocacy and even a bit of luck I was successful! Within the first few days, I seemed to be putting one fire out after another. My brother's adjustment was not easy and he was impatient, in pain and dependent. To him, nothing good was happening.

I knew that I could not leave him with the state of affairs as they were. On his first night, I stayed with him until after his dinner, which he did not like, and my plan was to go to my hotel room and get some sleep. When I tried to leave, my brother became agitated and angry with me and told me that I could not leave him there and if I did he would chase me out the door and hang onto the bumper of the car. I explained that I would be back in the morning and assured him that I would talk to the admissions director to see if they had a private room for him. It appeased him for the time being, but I knew that I needed to get him into a different room quickly. He was having a difficult time with making it to the bathroom, due to his physical weakness along with his loss of bowel control.

To top it off, his new roommate just stared at him and did not reply to anything my brother said. My brother, an outgoing person, tried to start up conversations, but because of the roommate's mental status, it was not going to happen. He told me that it bothered him every time he had to walk by the roommate to use the bathroom, because it was painful and he had issues with the process. I understood his complaints and agreed that I would do everything I could to get his room changed, if at all possible.

Cutting through the "Red Tape"

His Medicaid status limited the type of room he was eligible to have, so I knew that I might have some difficulty getting his room changed. I never told him this so as not to dash his hopes. I also felt uncomfortable in the room and the hall itself was very depressing. There were many long term people living in the wing where he was placed, and he realized this and it bothered him. It wasn't a place where people went to get better, but instead were there to be taken care of because they could not live independently. He was there to heal and get stronger in hopes of eventually getting better and going home to live independently once again.

The wing he was in scared him and depressed him even further, which clearly was not good for his own emotional well-being. When I left him that night, I vowed that I would get things figured out in the morning and I would do everything I could to get him moved. I reminded him that he could call me anytime during the night if he needed to talk.

Advocacy Mixed With Serendipity

I didn't waste a minute the next morning in trying to find the right staff member to talk to about moving him to another room, preferably with a closer bathroom and private. I realized that this was like asking for the moon, but my attitude was it never hurts to ask. In this case, I planned on hoping for the best, and at the same time I was cautiously optimistic. I found the Director of Admissions I had met the day he moved in. It was up to me to share with her that the room was not working out for my brother. I told her that he had told me that he hated his room and everything else about the place. Because I, too, was uneasy with his room conditions, I realized that his reactions were not just adjustment-based, but legitimate feelings and concerns.

I had to wait about twenty minutes until the director was free. I felt very fortunate when she invited me in to sit down and talk with her about my concerns. She listened very thoughtfully and to my surprise was open to the idea of moving him and even had a room in mind that had just become available after a long term resident had died that week. She explained that the room was very small, with a single bed and a bathroom attached. She offered to show it to me. I was so pleased at how very sensitive to my brother's needs she was. I tried to avoid complaining about my brother's situation, and instead tried to come from a place of concern and problem solving, not one of blaming (even though I felt like pointing out every single thing that was wrong since the day we arrived). It took restraint on my part, because I was so stressed by my brother's feelings and needs. However, once I knew I had the support of the director, I also explained that we had a problem with his pain medication due to miscommunication and a late order for his prescriptions. She agreed to look into this problem and was understanding and accommodating, to which I was very grateful. With her assistance, this problem was also solved. My advocacy was working but what I did not expect was the next series of events that led to my brother moving to a new room within an hour or so from my asking that he be moved. And, how it all came to be was nothing short of serendipity.

I never could have imagined how smoothly things went after I took action to ask for a new room. The most wonderful part of what transpired was that I first went to look at the room before we presented it to my brother. What I saw was a cozy, small room, with one twin bed and sunshine streaming brightly through the window. There was a bathroom within a few feet of his bed, so that he could make it by hanging onto things along the way. I hoped and prayed that he would feel as relieved as I did when he saw this room.

As the Director was showing me the way to the room she was considering, she saw the inspector, who was overseeing the facility's Medicaid compliance and said, that's exactly who I need to talk to about moving your brother. It was by luck that she was there on this day, as she only comes periodically for inspections. She introduced me to the inspector and told her about my brother's situation. She had a clipboard in hand and was very officious, but also seemed warm and understanding. I told her that the room seemed perfect for his medical needs. She then offered to go with me to talk to my brother. She wanted to hear from him directly and assess him herself before agreeing to apply Medicaid status to the room for compliance purposes. She also wanted to review his chart. After this interview and review of his current room, she suggested I take him to see the room and then let her know his feelings about it. He was so pleased to have someone listen to him and hear why the room was not a good fit for him. I felt like we hit the jackpot when this all fell into place.

The walk to the room was exhausting for him. I was amazed at how weak he had become. As we got to the threshold of the room, he took one look, smiled and said, "Can I stay here?" He then plopped down in the chair next to the door and said, "This is my room. Do I have to leave?" I told him to rest there and I would go tell the director of admissions that he liked the room and hopefully, he could stay there. The inspector/supervisor and the director both agreed that he could stay, because of his special medical needs and concerns that were not being met where he was placed. When I went back to tell him, he was lying on the bed with his eyes closed, looking as content as could be.

In this case, my proactive advocacy was effective, but another element added was some serendipity coupled with two administrators with heart, empathy and compassion. When I look back I often felt like I was drowning in a sea of red tape, understaffing, burned out staff, and needs I could not meet no matter what or how hard I tried. In this case, I felt success came with a combination of taking a risk, asking questions, finding the right people to talk to and presenting the situation from a place of honest concern. I stayed away from blame and kept a lid on my anger and frustration. And, to be sure, a little luck on that day went a very long way.

Once this room change happened, it opened the door to making my brother's time as comfortable as possible. The new room was at the end of a hall next to a visitors lounge. It made for a great place for me to go when he wanted privacy, or for him to visit with friends who visited him. Sometimes he wasn't up to getting out of bed, but when he was the option was not only there for him, but about ten feet from his door.

Another unexpected bit of luck was that a dear friend of my brother's, who lived near the nursing home, found out that he was moving to her area and she stepped up and offered to help. She visited him every night on her way home from work, and she spelled me so that I could go home to get my life in order and take a break.

One Problem Solved, More Problems Arise

In the beginning, my brother continued visits to the original oncologist, until the one hour trip to and from the hospital became far too difficult for him to tolerate. It seemed to me that the treatments were making my brother worse. I continued to feel that my questions were not being answered. It was decided to transfer all of his treatments to the center behind the nursing home. It was a brand new state of the art oncology treatment center, providing everything he needed. I was disappointed in the lack of information being given to me by the other center and was looking forward to getting some answers from the new oncology treatment facility.

A Turn for the Worse

One night, while in the nursing home his pain was so intense his friend took him to the emergency room and this is when they found lesions and tumors on his spine impinging on his spinal cord. Steroids were added to his medication, which increased his appetite but would not stop the metastasis of the cancer. Preliminary tests showed Osteolytic Metastasis. This led to treatment by radiation of his spine for pain and to ward off paralysis. I learned through reading, that the type of pain he experienced indicated possible metastases which meant he had an incurable disease. This is not what we learned or were told at the time. I found this out from my own recent research to better understand what happened to him.

Once the findings were in, I went with my brother to meet with the radiologist. This meeting was like something I had never experienced. The radiologist took a lot of time talking to him about his love of music and art and his talents. The doctor had the same passions and related very well to him and put both of us at ease with his personable and kind rapport. He did tell my brother that he had scheduled radiation of his spine to help reduce the size of some tumors found that were pressing on nerves and also preventing him from walking. He gently explained that there was some metastasis of the cancer, but he hoped the radiation would help. He also told him that he was not strong enough to go through chemotherapy at this time.

When they came to take my brother for radiation from his office, he took me aside and said to me with compassion and care, "This is not good. Don't change your Christmas plans, but there is no cure. He may live six months or a year, but of course nobody knows the answer to this except God." Radiation would be continued in an effort to shrink the tumors on the spine to try to "ward off paralysis." At this point, he was now in a wheelchair and the pain was excruciating with break through pain occurring often. It was time to call hospice to help with the management of his pain, provide emotional support and to supplement the nursing home with their oversight of my brother's needs.

Hospice Care

This time, I knew what to expect with respect to the evaluation for hospice services; however, my brother's response and reaction was very different than with my elderly family members. I tried to prepare him for why I thought hospice could help him. None of what I said was easy and he did not want to hear it. I reminded him of the many times that he called me in the middle of the night in excruciating pain, feeling helpless. I tried to explain that oftentimes patients do better with hospice oversight, when someone's pain cannot be helped. The idea of hospice would provide, "a belt with suspenders," to assist the facility where he was being cared for to provide what he needed to keep him more comfortable.

As I spoke to him, I felt like the grim reaper. He was very unhappy with my idea. I understood why completely, yet I felt strongly from my prior experiences that it was a good option. To him, it was a death sentence. I told him that I had arranged for the hospice social worker to come that day to explain what their services could do to help him. I did not push him but told him to think about it and we could talk about it after he rested. The social worker to her credit was not pushy at all and left him information about their services. I totally empathized with his fears and resistance. One of the first services offered was to meet the hospice Chaplain, which proved to be extremely helpful to both of us. We all prayed together. He was anxious to share our experience with my sister, as was I. This was a good way to help us both cope with the feelings associated with the need for hospice. The spiritual support proved to be very helpful.

The Gifts and Benefits of Music Therapy

Around the time that hospice was added to his care, my cousin's wife and colleague called to offer to play music for him in the nursing home. They were both studying the benefit of playing therapeutic music for patients to help decrease pain and to improve their well-being and offer comfort and support through the sound of their instruments; a string bass and flute. They were in the process of becoming certified music therapists, so this opportunity was a win/win for everyone.

My cousin's wife knew about my brother's situation, as I had been in contact frequently with her husband, my cousin, a physician's assistant, and big support to both of us from the beginning of my brother's health problems. His father was the pathologist who reviewed his initial pathology report. He and his family lived in the town where my brother had first been hospitalized and he helped us through support and knowledge. He also came to assist when he was initially brought in for his brainbleed.

On the day they selected to play, my nephew and his family were there for a visit and were able to join us to listen to the music. We could not fit everyone into his room, so we were given permission to use the lounge.

When I told my brother that they were coming, he told me he felt too sick and weak that day to leave his room. He had very little strength and was having great difficulty walking. I let him rest a bit and came back to check on him when everyone had arrived. I suggested I take him in his wheel chair to the lounge and he could stay as long as he could tolerate it. He agreed to give it a try.

Each piece of classical music they played was introduced with a story about who wrote the music, details about the composer and the style of music based upon the time it was written. The first piece happened to be one my brother knew well and liked. He nodded his head and said, "One of my favorites!" From this point forward he sat, with his eyes shut, soaking in the beautiful sounds and clapped at the end of each piece played. My four-year-old great nephew, also listened quietly for most of the concert and yelled out at one point, "I want to learn how to play like that." There's nothing like comic relief to add some levity to a very somber time in our lives.

I remember my brother smiling with his eyes shut most of the time they were there, soaking in the music and looking more and more at peace. He even made a comment or two about the compositions played. In addition, during the "concert," his energy and mood visibly improved. As a musician himself, this was the best medicine he could have had on that day. He was surrounded by beautiful music and people who loved him. And, a clear medical, physical and psychological benefit was that for approximately thirty-six hours or so after this experience, his need for pain medication actually diminished and a palpable calm came over him. He slept better that night according to his aide.

He talked about the experience many times later, as did I. This was a gift that kept on giving to all of us lucky enough to have been there that day. I so appreciated how much I benefitted as a family member from this therapeutic music opportunity. I still remember feeling a sense of calm come over me as I listened to the music and also watched my brother's facial expression change from distress and visible discomfort to a relaxed affect with a bit of a smile at times. The session lasted about forty-five minutes. The soothing melodic sound of their string bass and flute was truly powerful and therapeutic.

What I learned is that even during some of the darkest hours of caregiving there can be a glimmer of light and hope. We may not be able to stop the end of life from happening, but we can live each moment knowing that there are things we can do along the way that can have a positive and sometimes profound difference for those we are caring for. As in the case of the personal concert, I never would have thought music would make such a difference.

Final Two Holidays

I was able to leave to go home on Thanksgiving and Christmas and thankfully, each time dear friends were there to cover while I was away. I visited my brother in between each holiday. His last Thanksgiving was spent with friends, who were like family. This invitation was one met with apprehension because he was so ill. He had no appetite but getting out of the nursing home to be surrounded by friends, whom he loved and who loved him, was very important to him. The invitation meant the world to him, yet at the same time, I knew by his voice that it was a sad experience, because he could not enjoy it like he could when he was well. He had very little strength that night and I was told he stayed in one chair the entire time.

By Christmas time he was getting much weaker and going out was no longer feasible with the cold temperatures, snow and ice. So instead of visiting someone for Christmas, our friends offered to drive up to visit him. I was grateful that he would not be alone and that I would have a break to go home for a bit and be with my husband during the holiday.

My brother enjoyed these visits and expressed to me that he felt loved and that he was touched by people's level of caring. He mentioned enjoying laughing and reminiscing with old friends. I called during the visit and he gave me the blow-by-blow of what they did. It wasn't long after this visit that his health began to decline rapidly. By now, hospice was fully involved supplementing the nursing home services. It was determined that his medical needs would be treated through palliative care to keep him comfortable but not treat the disease with curative goals. Our hope that he would someday be strong enough for chemo therapy was no longer viable. The clock was ticking. I wished that I could turn back time and go back to better, healthier days. This turn of events was heart wrenching and painful, and very difficult to accept for everyone; family and friends alike.

Moving To a Hospice House

All hope for curative cancer treatment had ended. The health professionals could not predict when, but there was a consensus that short of a miracle, his cancer had advanced to the point of no possibility of remission or cure. We now had the option of a hospice house run by the same agency that came to the nursing home to manage his palliative care. One of the reasons I chose the hospice center that I did for my brother, was because of the continuum of care that they offered. If and when my brother needed to move out of the nursing home to receive twenty four hour hospice care, we learned that the agency that had been recommended had within the last year or so built a hospice house that one could only dream of for their loved one.

It turned out that the same person whose foundation had funded the oncology center where my brother received treatments had built the hospice house. It was state of the art, staffed by well-trained compassionate nurses and aides. All needs that should be considered in the development of this center, including what the family members needed as well as its patients, were addressed.

Although I wanted to be the one to show my brother the hospice house and help him to move, he refused to go with me, as he saw this option as a death sentence. I had no choice but to again reach out to my cousins, who had helped many times during his illness. This time they offered to go check the hospice house out, too, and then talk to my brother. They lived about two hours from where his nursing home was, which made things more doable for them, but nonetheless, their helping my brother and me during this time was amazingly helpful. They both had very busy lives of their own, but when they saw the need they came through beyond what I ever expected.

Thanks to the help of my cousin and his wife, my brother was successfully moved into the hospice house on a Friday when an opening became available and, although he was very scared, he agreed to go with them. My plan was to return the Tuesday after. My other cousin, who owns the family cottage, where everyone congregates each summer, asked if she could help out and go be with him in between my cousins moving him in and my being able to get back to be with him. She had kindly done this before since my brother became ill. Without this backup, I honestly could not, in good conscience, have left him alone. We still had our typical sibling squabbles at times, but they definitely diminished near the end. Petty things we argued about before became so meaningless. In the face of death, the small stuff becomes even smaller if not completely insignificant. The big stuff was just around the corner and it was worse than what I had imagined.

My cousin and I were close, but he and my brother were especially close. My cousin was younger than both of us and had lost his brother to a drowning accident at age twenty-one years. He also had just recently himself survived stage 3 colon cancer and was at this point only just over a year cancer free. I know from what he told me that any time he went into the hospital to visit my brother he was flooded by memories of his own experience and that it affected him deeply, which is very understandable. Not only had he just gone through similar experiences himself, but now he was there by my brother's side, knowing that his cousin would likely lose his battle against cancer.

I felt so grateful to have him and his wife's unconditional loving support. His wife stepped up a few times to drive him to an appointments when I was not in town. They also visited him on weekends. I asked my cousin and wife to please help move my brother into the hospice house while I returned home to Florida to get my life in order. They moved him the day after I flew home, which was a Friday. I would be back on Tuesday. In the meantime, my other cousin flew in to visit my brother until I could get back. I was able to stay in touch with him by phone. Regardless of this connection, I felt like I had abandoned him every time we talked. The conversations became shorter and shorter as he became weaker and weaker.

I sent out an update via email regarding where he had moved. People responded by supporting me, and also contacting my brother or sending him things; one of which were soothing musical CD's from our west coast cousins. This support was so heartening for me as well as for him. In addition to cards and calls, people stopped in if they were in the area to see him. On one of the last visits he had before he died, he was described as being funny and silly and had a burst of energy that they didn't expect to see at all. I know it's not easy to visit someone near death, and for someone to make a special trip to visit took some of the pain away.

Death Is Near

Death came too early and too quickly in my brother's life. And, although I had experienced being with my parents when their passing was near, as with almost everything, this time was different. Fortunately, I was given a booklet by the hospice center to read, which turned out to be very helpful to me leading up to my brother's passing. The booklet titled, "May I Walk You Home?" is a guide for hospice caregivers, provided by, Woodland Hospice House, Morey Bereavement Center, (Hospice) woodlandhospice.com/hospice.html. Within this site is some other very helpful free information. Such information helped me to better understand some of the behaviors and changes I saw in my brother. I was comforted by learning that what he was doing and experiencing was not abnormal. Again, knowledge is power, in the sense that the booklet information made me feel less afraid and more in control of my feelings.

A few specific examples with my brother that happened was that a couple of weeks before he passed, while visiting him, he asked me if I saw the two figures in the corner of his room? I looked and saw nothing. He told me they have come to see him a few times. I asked him questions, such as, "do they say or do anything?" And, his response was, "No!" Yet, he went on to explain that he knew they were there for him. I wondered if they were angels based upon his description of them. They were not scary he said, just present in the corner. He wished that I could see them, too.

Another example of what the booklet suggested may happen preceding death, was an experience our friend, Bob, had with my brother when he visited him. My brother suddenly had increased energy and a goal to go to work. At this point, my brother was using a wheelchair most of the time. When Bob walked in, my brother rose out of his bed, dressed himself and told him, "I have work to do." Mind you, at this point, he had only been able to ambulate with assistance or with a wheelchair. Once dressed, he started to walk down the long hall and said, "I have to get to work, I have work up there to do." Bob did not try to stop him, but walked with him to support him from falling. They walked all the way to the exit door. It was there that my brother stopped and realized he could not leave the building. My brother wanted to go to the place he loved and worked; the place (our summer home in Michigan) he visited every summer since he was young, and that had been the inspiration for much of his art and music. What I had read in the hospice booklet explained that it was not unusual before someone dies to exhibit this type of drive, energy and purpose and desire to "go on a trip."

One quote from the booklet describes what our friend witnessed. The booklet states: "Often a dying person will talk about traveling, about having to go away, to take a trip. He/she may say something simple like, "I've got to find my shoes," or something more detailed, such as "The train is coming," or "I've got to stand in line for the train." The method of transportation your loved one mentions may relate to things he/she liked to do during life: a motorcycle, a bicycle, a horse. "I want to go home" is very common even if your loved one is already home."

I also learned that a vision of something that appears to be an angel or figure of a person or people is something that is documented as happening to others prior to death. Knowing this helped me to understand that what my brother was seeing and talking about may not simply be a function of the medications he was taking. I still don't fully understand the phenomenon, but knowing that it is common and not unusual was reassuring and comforting.

I did see changes in energy with all five of those I cared for before they died. The level and type of energy is expressed differently by each person, but there was a definite shift in energy and purpose. For my father, he talked all night long before he died. Each person showed signs of some improvement or more energy as death became closer.

Soon after my brother was successfully moved into the hospice house by my cousins, I flew up to be with him in his final days. Upon arrival, I felt physically ill. I can't recall the exact sequence of events, but this is what I can remember. As I walked into the hospice house I was kindly escorted to my brother's room by a staff member. The name of the room on the door had a plaque with a name in memory of someone with the same first name as our mother. I recall that being comforting to me. My cousins greeted me and came out into the hall where we hugged one another in silence.

A Call from My Own Doctor

Before I could set foot in his room, my cell phone rang and it was my ear, nose and throat doctor from Florida calling with results from a test I had back in November. It was now late January. He asked me, "Is this a good time to talk?" I told him that I had just arrived to walk into my brother's hospice room where he was dying from cancer. He remembered I had told him of my brother's cancer at my visit in the fall, because the reason I had gone to see him in the first place was based on my brother's strong urging that I have my "hoarseness" checked. My brother and I had talked over the phone so often that he noticed a change in how I sounded. I attributed it to exhaustion from travelling and stress and the fact that he'd call me day and night, and sometimes it woke me up. He wouldn't accept my rationale and said to me, "Look what happened to me by ignoring symptoms. You have to promise me you'll go to the doctor!" I had gone for an appointment back in November, where a scope of my throat discovered that my right vocal cord was paralyzed. My doctor then ordered a CT scan of my "head and neck."

It was now the third week in January and I had never heard back from the doctor or his office with my CT scan results.

Typically, I would have called to check on what the findings were, but at this point with everything going on in my life, I figured no news was good news. As it turns out, my doctor had his own health emergency and had been off work and had not seen the test results until that day. This call was to tell me the findings of this test. He said, "I am sorry I didn't call sooner, but I was out for a kidney stone myself and just got back to work! I do not like what I see on the results of the scan. I have you scheduled for a PET scan for this Monday at 10:00 am. This test needs to be done as soon as possible. The timing of this and the report itself was upsetting but honestly, with my brother dying of cancer my attention was on him, not me. I did tell the doctor that I was scheduled to fly back on Sunday night and if that went as planned I would go have the PET scan on Monday. At this point, I needed to go into my brother's room, tell him I was there and hold his hand.

Before me was my dying brother. Hours beforehand, he was able to say a few words in response to a call I made to him telling him that I had landed in Detroit and Bob had picked me up and we'd be there shortly. His answer, "Good." By the time I actually got to his room, he was still able to lightly squeeze my hand back in acknowledgement of my being there but he could no longer speak and did not open his eyes. That was the very last time I got any noticeable response from him, but this I learned did not mean that he didn't know that I was there.

It was on a Tuesday late afternoon when I arrived. My cousins, who had moved him into his hospice room the Friday before, were able to come back to be with us when I came back into town. We took turns going to his bedside to soothe him, hold his hand and talk to him. He was no longer able to respond, although I knew he could hear us. The room was very large and afforded everything we needed. My cousins left that evening after we ate and had some wine together in my brother's room. Bob stayed there through my brother's death.

Sleeping in My Brother's Hospice Room

If someone had told me that one day I would sleep in a room in a recliner, with my brother in a bed next to me dying, I would never have believed it. Yet when the hospice support staff offered this option to me I agreed to do it. My brother's friend also slept in the room on a pull out couch. I lay awake listening to my brother's labored breathing and do not recall doing much sleeping at all. I remember frequently leaving the room and noticed Bob sleeping well. The experience was very uncomfortable emotionally and physically. I wanted to run away, but I also wanted to be there and tell him I was there for him. My head was filled that night with memories, regrets and thoughts of the future without him.

Something I learned from my experience with my mother, is that as hard as it may be, we need to let a person go when it is their time to die. This means letting go of our own need to keep them with us. I can't fully explain this, but I have now witnessed it a few times. In my brother's case, his buddy could not let him go. Without going into detail here, a nurse finally ushered him out of the room so I could have some quiet time with my brother in his final moments. I could hear my brother's music playing throughout the hospice house. I was so touched by the fact that the staff did this for us. They knew death was very near and they were honoring his life. I stood by my brother's bed and told him that his memory would live on through his art and music. I thanked him for being such a good brother to me. In retrospect I feel so lucky to have had this opportunity to say goodbye despite how deeply heart wrenching it was.

Facebook

Facebook had always been a point of contention between us. And, on this night of saying my final goodbye I told him that he was, "Right about Facebook and that now I can see why it had been so important to him and why he yelled at me to start using it about a year or so before he became sick." I also told him that I would make sure that the information about him would be sent to all his friends on Facebook. Bob would help me," I told him.

His Last Breath

At around 2:30 a.m. as with my mother, I left his room to use the restroom. I told the nurse where I was going, so she went and checked on him within a minute or so of my leaving the room. While in the bathroom crying, the nurse knocked on the door, and said, "He is gone." I ran to the room and remember that when I saw him, I saw a bright light flash before me. I doubled over in grief and could barely breathe. His belabored breathing was no more and the fluid leaving his body had stopped. To say that I was surprised just doesn't cover the emotions I felt. I knew he was dying and it would happen any minute, but when it happened it was as though I never knew the end was near. Intellectually and logically yes, but emotionally and physically it was as though it was something I just found out, without any forewarning.

The nurse was by my brother's side, and then Bob came into the room. He tried to comfort me, but I did not want to be touched or seen by anyone. I actually physically pulled away from him and ran to the meditation room. I wanted to be alone and cry alone. I remember putting a blanket over my head, so as to shut out the world around me. The male aide that had been so compassionate with my brother came in and squatted at the foot of the couch where he found me under the blanket. He talked to me, with so much kindness and understanding. He just touched my foot and told me he was there for me if I needed anything at all. I told him that I needed to call my sister. His presence helped me to get it together to get my cell phone and dial her number. He thoughtfully left the room when I dialed and reached her. She answered on the first ring. She knew by my earlier update that death was imminent. I could barely finish my words and cried while we talked. My sister, as always, was strong and supportive.

After hanging up, I had about two hours of fitful sleep. I was asked to sign some papers to release my brother to the funeral home right after he died. We had made all the arrangements ahead of time with the local funeral home so I didn't have too much to worry about. As I walked down the hall after going to sit in my brother's room after he had been taken away to the funeral home, Bob stopped me to tell me what he thought should be done next. I know he meant well, but I could not deal with anything like this at that moment. I told him such and I went back into the meditation room and shut the door. I honestly don't know where he went after this. In retrospect I felt badly about being so abrupt with him, but honestly when we are faced with such grief anybody can act differently than they typically would. Someone else may react differently.

I recall telling Bob that it was okay to post on Facebook that my brother had died. This led to a friend coming to attend the in-house memorial service for family and staff. She brought her dog whom she had brought to my brother when he lived in the nursing home. She also brought a very good friend of hers, whom I also knew. I remember feeling that I really wanted the service to include just my cousins and our friend and staff who wanted to come. I reacted in a way that I don't think I would have done normally. My cousin also wanted it to be just family. We consulted with the Chaplain who helped us process the acceptance of them being there. We didn't ask them to leave, but I remember again this need and feeling of wanting privacy coming over me so strongly.

Family Comes Through Again

My nephew and his family got a room in my hotel. Their support was more than helpful to me. One thing we did together was swim in the hotel pool. Being with the kids was revitalizing and was so helpful to me during this very dark time in my life. I felt so fortunate to have them with me and will forever remember this time spent together as we grieved and planned regarding details for what would come. My then four-year-old great nephew was particularly effected by the loss of my brother. He and my brother were "two peas in a pod." They had a very deep connection. I still have such great photos of their silly playful games together during their summer visits up north. My brother had a way of making anybody laugh, and his childlike imagination sparked the joy in kids and adults alike. Memories like this are what keep him alive in my heart and mind.

Our Chaplain Connection

Once my brother was under hospice care in the nursing home, a visit from their chaplain was offered if he chose to meet her. As a family member, I, too was given the option to talk with the chaplain, which I opted to do. We both liked the chaplain and stayed connected through his passing and I after his death. She reminded us of our sister, actually. This connection was so important for both of us. Together we gathered strength from the power of the prayer and human comfort from the minister. I remember all of us holding hands while he laid in bed, so helpless and I can only imagine so frightened by the unknowns that lay ahead.

The chaplain was there for us after my brother's death as well. She visited us in the hospice house and this is when I asked her if she would do a memorial service when the time came for us on site in the Meditation Room. She explained the process and agreed to do it. I was grieving deeply but also trying to organize things and do my part in taking care of my brother, too. We were able to hold a small service the morning after his passing. My cousin and his wife, and Bob and two friends of mine attended. We cried and prayed. In the background, we played a song from my brother's CD. My cousin put his arm around my shoulder during the short memorial. I remember how comforting that gesture and physical connection felt. We then used the hospice house kitchen to break bread together. I could not stop shaking and could not eat. On the one hand, I wanted to hide and be alone, but on the other hand I gathered strength from people being there with me. This was Friday; I would not go home until Sunday.

My brother was a fighter and did not leave this earth easily. It was a painful slow process to watch and although at some level I am glad I was there for him, I also wish I could have remembered him healthy. I have found since then that I do have the good memories of him and have been able to leave the end of his life behind. It was difficult, painful and something I would not want anyone else to go through. I now focus on how lucky I was to be there for him in his time of need. And, for this I am very grateful.

CHAPTER SEVENTEEN

MY FINAL THOUGHTS

From the point of my brother's diagnosis and all that happened between that time and his untimely death, my sense of time was altered. Sometimes, time seemed to go really fast, but what stands out most for me, is that my time spent overseeing his care felt like an eternity. These were the longest six months of my life. And even though I had external support, I felt incredibly alone. On the one hand, I wanted to be with people, but on the other hand I felt like a burden to others. I had a difficult time shifting away from my worries about my brother and my internal tug of war around wondering should I stay or should I leave each time I needed to return home. I went to social events and felt guilty for enjoying myself, which pretty much undid any joy. I wanted to be with people but also felt like retreating.

The hardest times were whenever my brother was faced with another brain surgery. I would make the four hour journey to be with him for support and sit in the surgical waiting room alone. I never asked anyone to come with me and honestly, I didn't have the energy to ask anyone, nor did I want to sit and talk with anyone. Sometimes I called people, or texted, but no matter what, I still felt so alone and helpless.

I was stunned at how my time with my brother seemed to stand still. I attribute it to what we were hoping for, waiting for, wanting to happen or not wanting to have happen. When things in life are fun and we don't want the time to ever end, time flies by. Kind of like when you're a kid on summer vacation. When in school, the year seemed to last forever, when summer break came, it flew by. Another example was waiting for Christmas as a kid; it seemed like an eternity. As an adult, we still have the same phenomenon with time lapse. And I think most caregivers would agree, that being by the side of someone who is terminally ill can feel too slow, or too fast depending on which side of things we are, that is pre or post-passing. No matter what, my sense of time was definitely affected each and every day.

Our Final Farewell

My brother had told me a few months before he died to "Have a big party when I am gone!" So, that's what we did. He died in January, but we waited until July, so that we could have the "party" my brother wanted, where people could gather together to celebrate his life. We didn't talk about where he would like it held, but I decided with input from my sister that we would have the memorial celebration of his life at his favorite place near our summer home, at a golf course that our family had been a part of for over a hundred years. Friends and family came from near and far. My nephew played my brother's guitar and sang a song he wrote back in 1970 about the island he "loved so well!"

The minister from the church I attended in the summer, officiated a short service, and friends were given the opportunity to talk about my brother and their reflections around their relationship with him. It was beautiful. After these eulogies, my nephew played my brother's guitar.

Tears and laughter could be seen and heard and, as we listened to the song, I knew that this is what he would have wanted. Someone commented that they thought they saw him on the roof of the clubhouse looking down on all of us. It was a powerful remembrance and tribute to a life cut too short, but a life that left a legacy of art and music behind, as well as many people who loved him!! The thing I take away from this experience is the depth of feelings and the way people came through when times were tough.

A Ray of Sunshine

A source of happiness was that my brother's CD of songs was ready for his Memorial. We were able to listen to the album during the memorial celebration. The timing of this for my brother and all of us was bittersweet. I couldn't help but think about how driven he had been to complete this project and I wondered if at some subconscious level he knew his time was limited. One of his song titles was "Give Me Time!" My nephew and his wife produced an audio/video montage of photographs with my brother's songs playing through the celebration of his life. I sang and cried with friends as we supported one another in our loss.

Unfortunately, due to delays with getting things done with the company who would make the CD's, my brother never saw the actual CD and cover we had produced professionally. We all wanted him to see it, and hold it. This remains one of my biggest regrets. Fortunately, we did get it produced and were able to have many copies made and gave them to friends and family at his memorial service and to anyone else who wanted them.

Searching For the Good

When bad things happen to good people, I tend to search for reasons for why something bad has happened to someone who didn't deserve it. In this case, I recall that many of us who loved my brother found some solace knowing that his music and art would live on no matter what happened, which meant his memory would stay alive.

Losing My Brother Was the Hardest

Each time someone whom I was caring for died, it was difficult and affected me in different ways. My brother's death was the most difficult, primarily because of his age and all of the twists and turns related to his needs and health concerns. Everything seemed more urgent and more stressful along the way. As a long distance caregiver, I never felt like I did enough or was there enough. With time, I have been able to accept that I did all that I could and that I can move forward knowing that although it was a very difficult time in my life, I know I did what I could to help him. Would have, could have, should have, is an unhelpful exercise in futility and does nothing to remove feelings of grief. Grief and loss are part of life. Hard, yes, but with support, manageable.

How I Found Support along the Way

My brother and I were raised with religion and a belief in God; however, neither he nor I were big on going to church after we left home. My sister, being a minister, was there for others in their time of need. She also helped my brother and myself at times, especially with the feelings of anger that come with a situation where we felt out of control and unable to stop what was happening and our anger was expressed toward God.

For me, reconnecting with church after years of not being involved in an organized religion came in response to the loss of my parents. It was something I recognized in myself that I needed. What became most important during this time was the benefit of the relationship I had developed with the congregation's minister and his wife, now that I faced my brother's cancer diagnosis. I knew that the minister and his wife had met my brother a few times. They had shared with me that they admired his gift for music and art and told me that they often talked to him when he was painting in front of the gallery near their parsonage. No, my brother never went to their church, but this didn't matter to the minister at all. This connection ended up giving us both a very helpful and important source of support. I remember our talking about how fortunate we were to have them in our lives.

The day I received the call from my brother about the plan for his treatment, I was in town having lunch with a colleague and friend I used to work with. Our lunch was interrupted by a call from my brother. He had just been given the details of his radiation schedule and was completely overwhelmed by the news. I told him I couldn't talk but would call him in about fifteen minutes if that was okay, which I did. I still was not in a convenient place to talk but opted to walk while talking to my brother. This talk couldn't wait. I sensed his sense of urgency and understood his need. He started by telling me that I had to come back down to help him. I cannot remember all the details of what he needed from me, but I recall the feelings associated with his phone call and the good fortune and support that came together while I was on the phone with him.

Interestingly, I found a place to sit in the shade in front of the gallery where his paintings hung. And, although people were walking by and the street noise was loud, it seemed like the right place to be at the time. I was very focused and tuned out the world until I noticed my minister's wife walking toward me. She saw the look on my face and immediately sensed that something was wrong. She stopped walking and I shook my head and mouthed the words, "my brother!" She stopped and waited. When I hung up I stood up and she immediately hugged me and listened to my news and offered prayers and continued support any time I needed someone to talk to, which I took advantage of more than once. I will never forget her kindness and empathy. My brother connected with the minister, as did I, but I also had the added benefit of having occasional talks with his wife, who had a counseling background. She was an enormous help to me. The minister was too far away to visit my brother, so he called him. And, they both sent us supportive cards along the way. This was a huge source of support, as we faced the scary diagnosis of cancer.

A Life Coach Connection

Fortunately, due to a bit of serendipity, I was able to find an answer to how I would find the time to better take care of myself, become more pro-active and less reactive. As luck would have it, just over a year before my brother was diagnosed with cancer I met a "Life Coach" through a mutual friend. We were introduced because of the fact that at that point I had two published children's books and she had just published a book for cancer survivors. She herself had survived cancer and had developed a supportive program called, "What's Next for My Life".

When we first were introduced we immediately hit it off and began talking about what she had just published, and I told about my two children's books. From there she told me that she was a "Life Coach." Despite my own professional background as a social worker, I didn't know much about this particular helping modality/profession called "coaching." I wanted to learn more about what she did and how it worked. With this, she invited me to her house for a free "coaching session." I was moving in two weeks to northern Florida, so we used this life event for the session. I didn't know where our move and new life-path would take me and I welcomed the idea of having a free opportunity to learn more about life coaching, which also gave me an opportunity to explore what was "next for my life."

My mother had died less than a year beforehand, and I was embarking on a new journey in a new environment. I was excited yet apprehensive as anyone might be. Moving, like any new beginning comes with opportunity, adventure and some anxiety about what lies ahead. And, one thing I had been struggling with at the time was that I had put some of my personal goals on hold while caring for my family members and was trying to get my life ambitions/goals back on track.

After this one sample session, I did not sign on for anymore coaching sessions, but the two of us stayed connected on a professional level. I did leave with a sense that the coaching approach could be quite helpful and I enjoyed the experience. I gave her my books and she placed me on her professional email database, where I would receive informational emails for cancer survivors and family members. At this point, nobody I cared for had cancer, but I thought the resource could be helpful to others. Although I wasn't working as a social worker at the time, I gathered helping resources, as I always had to share with others if I saw a need, or someone asked me for help as a friend. It turned out, I ended up needing the help myself not too long after I had my own coaching session.

As a result of this earlier connection, I fortunately received an email from the life coach at the end of November in 2010, announcing a teleconference for family members of cancer patients. I distinctly remember reading the invitation thinking and hoping that this might be of help to me as I tried to support my brother's fight for life. At this point I was feeling completely overwhelmed and did not know where to turn. I quickly sent an email to the life coach and asked if she felt it I could benefit from calling in for support. She responded by suggesting that we first speak over the telephone. I recently found my emails with her and saw that they took place on December 1, which was when things were really turning for the worse for my brother.

This call to a "friend" shifted to a coaching session about half way through my telling her of my brother's situation and what I was most worried about. I know she heard my panic and deep distress about his situation and what it was doing to my own life. She stopped me and said, "Do you mind if I put on my coaching hat at this point?" I welcomed this offer and we continued to talk for about an hour. The call was so helpful I immediately felt the benefit of this telephone interaction. She offered coaching by phone, as she understood my schedule would be erratic and effected by my travel.

Coaching brought to me a new perspective, which helped lift the fog of long distance caregiving, along with the attached grief and loss. Our phone calls helped me to see things more clearly and realistically. The sessions helped to restore my sense of direction and empowerment. Coaching gave me knowledge, support, validation of feelings and gave me time to stop and look at things more differently and consequently more clearly. We can sometimes lose ourselves when we are in caregiver mode. And, although friends can help, they too can lose objectivity and may not be able to say the things we need or want to hear.

I considered traditional therapy, but realized I didn't have any time to set up appointments for myself because most of the time I was flying or driving in and out of town. I also considered getting involved in a cancer support group offered by the hospital, however, even that seemed too time consuming for me. Instead, I opted for the weekly one-hour phone sessions.

Coaching helped me find myself again. It reignited my inspiration, helping me to look inward and stop using my current life situation as an excuse to avoid my own personal goals. It helped me to take the risks necessary to get out of the quagmire of my situation. One big first step, was finding a new illustrator to finish the third book my brother was going to illustrate for me. I still have the e-mails where I shared what I would like the animal characters to look like, and his sketches he sent to me. I found another illustrator through a friend and the book was published in my brother's memory.

Coaching was like putting on a new pair of glasses and seeing clearly again. Today, I process and cope with things differently. I draw upon techniques I learned to manage my feelings and my life without being completely swallowed up by my situations. One important lesson: It is very difficult to be a good caregiver if we don't take care of our own needs, too.

EPILOGUE

It is hard to believe that it's been almost eighteen years since my first caregiving experience began, my most recent ending three years ago.

Like many of us, when the first "call" catapulted me into caregiving action, the role was foreign to me. The stressors associated with responding to family crises from afar opened my eyes to just how unprepared I was for much of what I would face. I quickly learned the importance of being a good advocate, skilled at finding resources and assistance for those I cared for and myself. I recognized that with each experience came different issues as well as commonalities. What I learned with one situation, changed from one hospital, nursing home, hospice agency or state. Each state, institution, facility and system had different ways of doing things from regulations, to support, to the care itself. And, of course there are the personalities of those providing care, services, support or advice. Like staffs and professionals, systems have different personalities, too. Such differences required learning and an ability to ask questions and for help from others. These differences extend to everything from medical care to business, real estate, and legal and facility oversight, end-of-life issues, and the list goes on.

With each family member, I learned that so much of our success comes from commitment and involvement. I dug deep with determination and a drive to help in every way I could. I armed myself with as much knowledge as possible, from talking to friends, family, going online, reading articles and books, or learning about each system where family received care or assistance. And, yes, there were times I felt like giving up! Those were the times I learned to reach out to others for support or to spell me.

I cannot tell you exactly what to say in each situation. Instead, I encourage you to find the right friend, professional, or someone within the system, such as a social worker, to help you find what you need and/or to accompany you.

One thing that proved most valuable was to find an ally within the system, be it a receptionist, supervisor, a particular nurse or aide, doctor, social worker, etc. During each one of my charges, I was successful in finding someone, giving me and even my family a sense of trust and support. Personalizing the relationship, by sharing my concerns and worries when not always being able to be on site or in the same town, increased my essential communication both with and from staff,

I learned to become a part of what I call the "communication loop of care," which included those who were involved in my loved ones care, be it anybody from a family member, an aide or the supervisor of the unit or floor they were housed. Since I could not be with them 24/7, I needed and wanted to remain present in some tangible way. Staff knowing I was interested and available made a marked and positive difference in overall care. We cannot always get everything that is needed, or that we think should happen, or even want, but by being available and present even from afar, the likelihood of good care for those we love is greatly increased. One word of caution, staff changes will mean that you may need to start over if someone leaves the system. My experience was that there is always someone on the inside or outside of the system who can help.

Since responding to my first family crisis, the amount of resources for caregivers has grown by leaps and bounds. There are websites, community support groups, caregiver support groups on Facebook, and many step-by-step tips for getting resources and information online and even via commercials.

As caregivers, we owe it to those we are helping to do whatever we can to help in a productive ways, such as by staying on top of resources and information and staying connected.

Some Helpful Websites for Me:

www.caregiver.com
www.thecaregiverspace.org
www.nextstepincare.org
www.whatsnextformylife.com
www.mayoclinic.org
www.agingwithdignity.org

www.nolo.com/legal-encyclopedia/helpin-seniors-manage-money-finances
www.theconversationproject.org
www.about.com/healthwoodlandhospice.com/hospice.html
www.bereavementnavigators.com

I am not recommending, but instead am sharing some of the websites that I referred to while caregiving and afterward. Websites change so by the time you may read this some may not exist. To find updated sites, you can search the web or ask others who have been caregivers.

Jacqueline Marcell's book, *Elder Rage—or Take My Father…Please!*, a book I happened upon during my first caregiving experience with my father, helped to normalize my situation. This book helped me realize that I was not alone and that other fathers with dementia behaved like mine. Marcell's experience helped me gain some insight that had been very difficult to achieve on my own. It was a lesson I carried with me to each caregiving experience thereafter.

My hope is that within my five personal stories, complete with successes and failures, you find some answers, support, validation and examples of what it takes to be supportive and successful advocates. One of my biggest realizations as a caregiver is that it is not a sign of weakness or failure to ask for help; it's a sign of courage and strength. I learned five times over that communication was the key to helping and even though I ultimately could not control everything, a most important lesson learned. And, yes, some of the best results came from serendipitous circumstances. But here realizing and benefitting from such serendipity depended upon being present as a caregiver, which is not always easy.

ACKNOWLEDGEMENTS

I am grateful for the encouragement and support of Reverend Vince and Molly Carrol.

I thank Dr. William Steele, for his coaching and encouragement to keep writing.

I thank my supportive husband, who helped me "keep it all together" while I provided oversight, care and unplanned response to crises over many years.

I thank my sister for her support and input and giving me breaks when needed. We were a good team! I also must thank my sister for giving me the "green light" to share our family stories.

My nephews, and their wives, gave "stepping up to the plate" new meaning when they received "my calls" for help.

I thank my cousin and his wife for their love and helpful support of my brother and me, whenever I needed a break or simply could not be there to sit by his bedside, or to take him to appointments.

I thank my cousin, and my aunt and uncle, for the times they checked in, offered to help when I was unavailable, or to visit my parents or brother. Their presence and positive support gave me peace of mind.

The list of friends who helped is too long, so at the risk of leaving someone out, just know that you know who you are and I and those who I cared for thank you then and now!

I thank Julliette for her attentive and kind care for my mother, giving our family peace of mind when we could not be there ourselves.

I am grateful to Paula Holland Delong for her Life Coaching during my darkest times of caregiving.

Lastly, I thank Dr. Patricia Ross, Editor/Publisher of Banyan Tree Press, for accepting my manuscript and publishing my book.

ABOUT THE AUTHOR

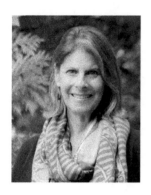

Caroline H. Sheppard's social work experiences include providing therapeutic clinical social work services to children and families in a Day Treatment Program and a Community Mental Health Center. Following her clinical experience, Ms. Sheppard worked as a School Social Worker.

In 1998, Ms. Sheppard's first book, *Brave Bart: A Story for Traumatized and Grieving Children,* was published. This story was inspired by her involvement with the Institute for Trauma and Loss in Children (TLC), while participating in their trauma and loss certification programs training, as well as a research project.

The author's second book, *Shadow Moves* (2003), addressed issues surrounding difficult and traumatic moves for children and her most recent book, *Brave Bart and the Bully* (2012), brings back the main character, Bart (a kitten in the first book), as an older and wiser cat who helps the kittens in his neighborhood with bullying. The books are currently published by Starr Global Learning Network/TLC.

Ms. Sheppard's career path changed when her parents needed her help. At the time, she was involved in a nonprofit children's organization as a volunteer. Once her caregiving from afar began, she never returned to her position as a school social worker.

Ms. Sheppard hopes that by sharing her own personal experiences with long and near-distance caregiving for five different family members over a fifteen-year period, coupled with the knowledge and insight gained from her professional background, her stories will help others when faced with similar challenges.

CPSIA information can be obtained
at www.ICGtesting.com
Printed in the USA
BVHW01s0507240218
508719BV00002B/179/P